The Mindful Corporation

The Mindful Corporation

Liberating the Human Spirit at Work

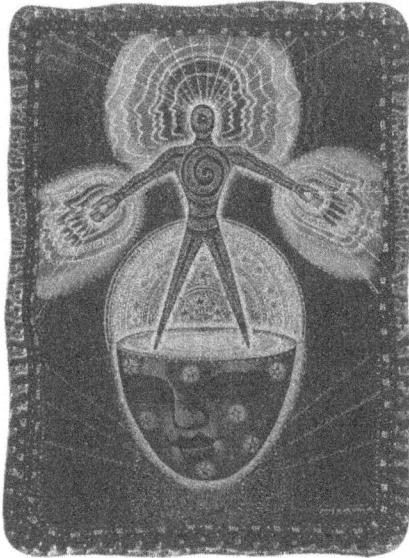

Paul Nakai / Ron Schultz

WIPF & STOCK · Eugene, Oregon

Resource Publications
A division of Wipf and Stock Publishers
199 W 8th Ave, Suite 3
Eugene, OR 97401

The Mindful Corporation
Liberating the Human Spirit at Work
By Nakai, Paul and Schultz, Ron
Copyright©2000 by Nakai, Paul
ISBN 13: 978-1-5326-9590-2
Publication date 7/7/2019
Previously published by Leadership Press, 2000

Table of Contents

Acknowledgements

The Mindful Corporation is meant to share many of our discoveries and insights in what we feel is one of the most impactful methodologies for positive change and improvement in business today. In writing this book, we have been fortunate in having the help and input of many people who have contributed in a variety of ways simply because we asked them.

From Senn-Delaney Leadership, we have enjoyed the support and encouragement of the senior management team and many of our colleagues throughout the organization. Larry Senn and John Childress embraced this idea of publishing our ideas and taking them to the world at large and have been willing participants and advisors in this great communication exercise. To both of them we owe our gratitude and appreciation for the opportunity to explore and access this thinking, and to grow and prosper. Jim Hart has provided great leadership in directing and supporting our efforts, providing us both cover when needed and insight whenever asked. He has been a well-spring of encouragement and an unparalleled strategic ally. Nick Neuhausel and Nitsa Lallas have both provided perspective and focus for our work, sharing their awareness and understanding to further our own.

Jim Ondrus, Jack MacPhail, Mike Marino, Yvonne Vick, and Rena Jordan have been nothing but incredibly supportive of our efforts, time and again giving us their feedback and appreciation for moving these ideas forward.

Within Senn-Delaney Leadership, Peter Brown has given us excellent advice and council on design issues. Esperanza Byrd has kept our efforts on line and coordinated. Penny Madden, Judy Gesicki, and Joan Goodwin have all helped us clear schedules, set up interviews, and facilitate a process that, in its complexity, can sometimes become overwhelming.

From an editorial and production perspective, John Cole has tirelessly and wonderfully designed this book and has been a consistent source of creativity and inspiration. Judith Blahnik helped us shape the manuscript and provided perspective that was invaluable in making sure we were as clear as we could be in describing what were often illusive ideas. In addition, Howard Sherman, a trusted mentor and a writing partner, offered continual reinforcement assurance, and clarification of ideas when the road got a little muddy. We would also like to acknowledge the efforts of Bonnie Norris and Ginger Levin who made certain the manuscript was in appropriate grammatical shape. And we'd like to extend a special thanks to Janet Rasmussen for taking our rambling conversations and transcribing them so accurately and faithfully, while continually assuring us that this formative process was actually leading somewhere.

We would also like to express our appreciation to Bob Gunn from Gunn Partners, Ron Adams, Bob Best from Atmos Energy, Larry Senn, Bob Pratt from the Volunteers of America, Bill Thompson from TVA, and John Horne from

International® for their insights and stories that have helped to enhance this book.

Ron Schultz

From a personal perspective, I, Ron, would first and foremost like to acknowledge my coauthor, Paul Nakai. From the moment we were introduced, we both knew there was a connection here that was important and valuable to us both. We write a great deal in this book about creating an environment in which we can access our wisdom. Paul has graciously and generously opened himself and his understanding to me in a way that has made the writing of this book possible, and has facilitated both of our abilities to tap into our source materials. I have learned a tremendous amount from him for which I am forever grateful.

I would also like to thank my wife Laura and my daughters Johana and Emily for being tolerant and patient while my focus was directed away from them. They are a constant source of goodness and wonder in my life, inspiration of the highest order.

Paul Nakai

In addition to the many dear colleagues and friends Ron has mentioned, I, Paul, would like to add my appreciation to the following people.

This has been my first attempt at writing a book and I truthfully don't know if there is another book in me. However, this would not have been possible without the coaching, effort, and reassurance of my coauthor, Ron Schultz.

I would like to add that these thoughts and insights would not have occurred without the patience and guidance of my more recent mentors and friends along the way. Robert Kausen, who introduced me to this path; Drs. George Pransky and Roger Mills, who have deepened my understanding over the past 19 years; Sydney Banks, who has made this awareness real; and Penny Rock, who, in the early days, assured me that these insights were not crazy possibilities for business.

I also want to acknowledge my mom, Miyako, and my sister, Cynthia, for always supporting me throughout my life.

And finally, the three people in my life who have never waivered in their belief in me, in spite of myself, have been my wife Nancy, my daughter Stephanie, and my son Johnathan. They have been my soul mates in this journey and I can never repay or express enough my love and gratitude to them.

Two Journeys Toward Understanding Thought

Mindful: Attentive, open to the possible, regarding with care, humbly observant

Paul Nakai

As a young man, when I looked out at the world, I honestly thought that I was viewing reality. I had heard about situations where a number of witnesses would view an event and each one saw something different, but I dismissed this idea and went through life with the attitude that the way that I saw things was the way they were.

I suppose that this attitude had its roots very early in my development as a young boy growing up in Hawaii. I remember trying to make sense out of life in order to learn how life worked, so that I could avoid the pitfalls and pains while enjoying the rewards and praise. I then went about discovering ways to affect, impact and change my surroundings, the situation, and the people in my life to better fit this vision. Perhaps that's the reason that I became an engineer…to learn the "laws" behind getting things to work. For a number of years, most of my efforts were directed in a selfish way to alter my circumstances with the belief that in so doing, I would be happier and more at peace.

I then extrapolated the philosophy behind the laws of physics to my interactions with people, as well as to how I would go through life. Much of my time was spent trying to make others happy or trying to avoid conflict. I dressed the right way or the way that I thought conveyed success and confidence. I hung around with the right people, lived in the right area, did the most currently popular things. I bought a home on the fashionable side of town, drove a Porsche, and played tennis. I took pride in the things that I had done or collected. What made this life so compelling was how real it seemed. After all, I could touch it, feel it, and drive it.

During this time, the most honest thing that I did was marry a woman whom I dearly loved and had wonderful friends and family who did not care about my idiosyncracies and quirks. More and more, I began to notice that there was a different feeling when I did things from the heart rather than based on what I thought I should do.

However, at the time, I did not realize how much a victim to my circumstances I had become. My external trappings of success and peace governed much of my actions, worries, and thoughts. Although things were going fine, in my quieter moments I was wondering if this was all there was. Was my life to be governed by making more money, having prettier trappings, and gaining more popularity or notoriety? And, what if I were to lose any of it?

Fortunately for me, my wife had learned about a program that seemed to have a dramatic positive influence on one of her friends. Through this course, I was introduced to another facet of life—thought and thinking. I knew that I thought, but I did not know what my thinking was at the moment. I was ignorant about its influence on my life. As I learned more about my thoughts, my relationship to this dimension became a mirror of my relationship to my earlier world of circumstances and events. I wanted to learn how to control my thoughts. I learned techniques to be more positive and to direct my thinking toward accomplishing more. After awhile, once again I began to feel like a victim. But this time it was to my thinking.

I could now explain the questions that existed in my previous level of awareness. But new questions started to appear. Although my life was a little less effortful and harsh than before, its was still stressful and full of judgment. Self-doubt and worry gave way to self-recrimination and tension. My intensity toward life was now directed toward understanding these principles of psychology. The tension and effort was focused both on the content of my thinking and on the quality of thinking habits that I had picked up along the way.

I hasten to add that it was also during this time that I noticed that I was becoming more and more comfortable with feelings like inspiration and non-contingent gratitude. I fell in "love" easier…and with people of all walks of life and nature. I noticed that I could see the grand beauty in life as well as in many people…tall, short, fat, lean, old, young, rich or poor. Many of my earlier friends thought that I had lost my competitive edge; my desire for the good things in life. When good things happened to me now, they explained it as just being lucky or "being in the right place at the right time." To them, I was living on borrowed time and any moment now the other shoe would drop. I was still happier than I had been before…but still, there was something missing.

About this time a good friend in one of the programs, offered me a job with his fledgling company. Originally, it was meant to be an opportunity to apply in the business community the "high performance" principles that I had learned earlier. However, within a few months I was introduced to another dimension of life that had an even more profound impact on my life than the first two phases. Through this understanding, many of the good ideas that I tried to live my life by became real. Morally, good ideas like "forgiveness" and "innocence," have taken on a real world perspective and pragmatic applicability to every facet of life. No longer are there separate rules for success in business, personal life, spirituality—or for being a parent, spouse, child or friend.

This most recent step has introduced me to and made real the source of thought, not just thought itself. As we explain throughout The Mindful Corporation, this is the difference between what we think and the fact that we think. This dimension is effortless and graceful and is the source of all of the wonderful traits and characteristics we attribute to being human; that is, being able to keep our bearings in all times, joy, wisdom, common sense, compassion, humor and contentment. It is the split moment before we recognize our thinking—our headwaters of inspiration.

I sometimes chuckle to think what my older friends must think of me today. Have I gone over the "edge," dedicated my life to a more thoughtful lifestyle, and forsaken all tangible things of this life? Far from it. This is a darn good life and one I mean to live. We don't have to go to a mountaintop to feel this way or spend each night in a sensory deprivation chamber. It is available to us whether we're giving a speech or doing the year-end accounting.

I feel as though I only have part of one foot on this path. At times I feel the grandeur and beauty of life, and at others, the pain and insecurity. I am learning to appreciate both as parts of life. Am I perfect or have I messed up since then? You bet! I've screwed up in the biggest ways, and these "wake-up calls" help put me more firmly back on the path to learn more about life, not just about me. I have had brief moments of insight when I have experienced this greater understanding behind life. I have come to realize more clearly that when things go "bad," it's because I step away from this source and into a game of my own making.

This is especially true and easy to do in business. The rules are so enticing to follow and they seem to make perfect sense. However, frequently it's not the behavior and actions that are in question. We can run the business with the spirit of contribution and service and still do what is necessary to make the business successful. Through this spirit, coaching is done in a mutually constructive manner, initiatives are smoothly implemented, discipline of action reinforced, change happens, and results get measured. This spirit and our innate sense of conscience can provide the guidance and direction we need to follow as long as we listen.

Three principles of life have been exposed to me. There are many others who are more articulate than I about these principles, but here is my understanding and experience as of this date:

1. One of the principles is the gift that we've been given to experience Life through our senses. I sometimes lose sight of this gift and take it for granted. At the very least when I am feeling down, I label the events

of Life as good or bad depending on my experience and expectation. Yet I am reminded that frequently individuals first see this gift on their deathbed when they come to realize that they will miss everything about life—not just the good stuff. Our capacity to experience Life and our ability to make things real is the gift. As we relax, this gift develops. As far as I can see, there are an infinite number of levels through which we can experience Life. It is a part of our journey both now and in the future. It is part of the Presence of Life.

2. Another principle is thought. As mentioned earlier, not what we think but that we think. This process of thought is the vocabulary through which our finite being communicates with the innate and infinite. To the degree that we can see this principle as that simply is the degree to which we can access the potential available to us without having to control or manipulate our thinking. It is our conduit with reality. The joy and insight we seek is readily available on the other side of the content of our thoughts. Thought is our experience of the present in action.

3. The final principle is that there is a transcendent intelligence out of which all life emanates. I have spent so much of my life looking for the truth, the rules to right living, the "source" of things, that I limited it by looking for something with boundaries and conditions. It was when I had an insight that in truth everything around me is present—that it is all around me and of me—that I had an experience of

the grandeur and universality of the present. It is the potential for everything that we seek and then some, and is always there. I discovered that one does not learn about the present, nor do we find it in special places. The present is not uncovered: It is owned.

I had spent so much of my life searching for the answers that I missed living Life itself. This was and still is my life yet I so enjoy the intensity of the beauty of Life. It is the feeling that I had the very first times that I held my daughter and my son. It was the calm sense of oneness I had when I viewed the sunset the evening my Dad died and knew that his spirit was still there. No sadness, just appreciation and awe.

Our intent with this book is that the thoughts contained herein not only make sense but also open a door in our minds for us to step through. But it is not the thoughts that are the end product of this writing. Our plan is to make each of our experiences of the present real, not just believe that they might be.

Ron Schultz

I grew up in a family in which consciousness was highly valued, but tended to be something one discovered through arduous introspection or painfully unearthed. I had never considered that it might be something I already had. I had felt its stirrings, but always associated those early rumbles with my hard work and willingness to "dig down." I remember sharing thoughts about my personal connection to my consciousness with some people who I felt close to and whose "intelligence" I trusted. My revelations were not well received, and to my thinking at the time, were belittled and devalued. I felt embarrassed and diminished for having revealed this part of me, in both my own and their eyes. Being no one's fool, I quickly put a policy in place that would safely hide away my, for want of a better word, "inner knowings."

Unfortunately, in closing down this part of my life over the years, I became cynical and incredibly judgmental of others who revealed similar drives for understanding and quests for meaning. At the same time, I was, of course, unable to keep my own thinking about these issues quiet. But rather than proceed along the more inward route toward understanding, I sought out the advice and ideas of famous scientists who could provide "real" knowledge about our understanding of the nature of the universe. Fortunately, as a journalist, I was usually able to find someone who would pay me to go and interview these famous people, which would then allow me a few minutes to pose to them the questions I really wanted to ask. In speaking to one Nobel Prize winning physicist who had discovered what we considered to be most fundamental about the universe, I put forward my proposition. I had this notion that somewhere in what he knew about fundamental matter there had to exist a spark of "true" understanding. We could then somehow build back up the ladder from that spark and prove that understanding and, ultimately, meaning existed. I was told rather unceremoniously that the bridges I was trying to build could not possibly be built.

As I became more frustrated in my attempt to seek outer confirmation for these more "spiritual" thoughts and perceptions, I closed down this side of my life to those I encountered even more. My wife, who bore the brunt of my cynicism and endured my increasing judgments about the folly of others' thinking in this arena, finally could take no more. She gave me an ultimatum. It was a painful wake-up call. What she was demanding, however was nothing short of my owning what I had always known, but had chosen to inter. This was skillfully reinforced by patterns of thinking I quickly and effectively had made habit.

Change or lose it all. It was an incredibly scary place to find oneself, until I discovered that what was being demanded of me was to do nothing more than to change into what I already knew. In building and rebuilding my relationships, I had to reopen myself, which meant that when I was confronted by a situation in which I had previously responded with cynicism and judgment, I needed to somehow react differently. The old patterned responses would no longer support me. I would eventually learn that what had kept me from changing was my thinking, which translated into my pride, and my concern about what others thought of me. But when the choice was between losing what I loved most or letting go of what I thought others might think of me, the choice was easy. The realization that followed was simple. When I allowed the outside world to hold down what I felt inside, I was unhappy and I made all those around me unhappy, too. I also discovered how releasing myself from this hold really meant digging out from the weight of the life bunker I had built. I was amazed how quickly those deeply fortified walls came crumbling down.

When I brought this way of being into the business world in which I worked, there were those who quickly judged and dismissed it. I recognized their mistrust as being just like mine. That's when I also realized how remarkable it was that we had all gotten to the same place of judgment and dismissal from so many different directions. It followed, then, that if we shared this negative reaction to the world, we shared the positive space as well.

It was shortly thereafter that I heard Hatim Tayabi, then CEO of VeriFone, speak about his experience in building his company into the powerhouse it had become. He began his talk by quoting the Zen master Shunryu Suzuki about the need to cultivate the "beginner's mind." Afterwards, I approached him and commented that it sounded like he was suggesting that in order for businesses to survive in this new globalized work world, we needed to create more mindful corporations and employees. And if that were true, were we ready for it? Tayabi's response was a surprising "Not yet."

A number of years after my encounter with Tayabi, I was introduced to a company, Senn-Delaney Leadership, that was actually trying to live these ideas and put them into practice. It was working with people in organizations to help them understand that the power and quality of their thinking could either limit or enable their growth. And they weren't delivering this message to small upstart companies, but to those within the Fortune 1000 that recognized, too, that they had to change or lose it all. It didn't take long for Paul Nakai, a long-time partner in Senn-Delaney Leadership, and me to decide that the time had come for The Mindful Corporation.

We realized that we all come to this place seeking deeper and more successful ways of understanding from a wide variety of experiences, opportunities, and directions. Our purpose in presenting the ideas contained within the Mindful Corporation is to share our thinking, and that of some of those with whom we have worked, and to shine a light on the nature of that thinking that either keeps us stuck where we are or liberates us to attain deeper and greater happiness and success. For as many have said before us, "We are just one thought away from making things different."

The Mindful Corporation

Chapter One

The Complex Mind-filled World

"In the beginner's mind there are many possibilities, but in the expert's there are few."

—

Shunryu Suzuki

Mindfulness is not a prescription for health. It is a journey toward realizing the health we already possess. The sooner we are able to recognize it and act out of it, the quicker we'll be able to react to our rapidly changing business environment, and therefore increase efficiency and productivity, and improve the lives of all who work within our organizations. Sound impossible? Perhaps it's time to explore health.

The Search for Fulfillment

Most people would admit that what they're looking for, both personally and professionally, is a lasting sense of fulfillment. How we go about attaining it is an indication of our understanding and health. If we live our lives seeking an outer fulfillment to satisfy our inner need, we may find temporary satisfaction in such things as achieving our goals, making more money, having possessions, and advancing upward. The problem with such external sources of fulfillment is that what we experience from them is short-lived. We see evidence of this in people who have achieved and are constantly driven to achieve more, people with possessions who desire even more possessions, and people compelled by ambition never comfortable in their current place in the world. This does not mean to imply that any of these things are bad. We're simply saying that many people try to quench their inner desires from an external reservoir.

We have found that as long as we seek fulfillment from the outside, we never satisfy our inner need for it. We go outside, for the most part, because we live our lives from a mind-filled perspective, and we externalize because we do not understand internalization. When we say "mind-filled," we are actually describing the clutter of unnecessary things we keep readily in mind—worry, stress, insecurity, pressure, anger, resentment, and all their attendant entanglements. All we can do from this cluttered vantage point is misdirect the mind. We then provide it with even more places to become stuck, and we therefore become more even mind-filled. The answer to this distracting continuum lies in our ability to see life as an inside-out phenomenon rather than outside-in. This is often a terrifying step for some people to take. So terrifying, in fact, that pain and unhealthful distraction are easier and more familiar choices.

When we are in this mind-filled state, we are less available to the present moment, less available to make clear decisions. This does not mean we are incapable of relating to others. We can learn certain rules, mannerisms, and techniques that help us live productive and contributing lives. These rules may be seen as indicators of levels of health or may provide a sense of direction. On the other hand, they may become rigid and inflexible ways to judge others and ourselves.

Sometimes, we find ourselves in a difficult place where we can't see any direction available to us. Every choice seems to be the same…bad. This, too, is an indication of the quality of our thinking. So what are we supposed to do? The mind-filled answer is look harder, work harder. The mindful answer is to stop trying to find a solution if a solution is not evident within a few seconds. "But we have to have an answer and we have to have one now!" If every choice looked the same to someone operating from a mindful perspective, it would be a signal to them to let it go for the time being and trust that the capability and capacity to find the right solution will emerge. It does, but not when pressed to do so.

Mindfulness is the ability to allow our minds to be open and uncluttered so we can see more clearly. When such things as stress, pressure, and worry cloud our vision, we filter our perceptions through lenses defused by these factors. Mindfulness emerges unfettered, without preconception or predisposition, and we all have access to it and its clarity. It may take a walk up a favorite trail or even a walk away from the conference table to come forward. How many executives have the courage to take that walk when hard-pressed to deliver? And yet, how often have we heard, "I get my best ideas in the shower, or while I jog." It is while the mind is given a rest that it responds with something new.

Going back and examining where we are stuck in our thinking won't help either. That tends to put us into an even more self-conscious role. The more self-conscious we become, the less free we are, and our propensity then is to move in the direction of mind-filledness instead of mindfulness. We are making the distinction here between thought and the place from which thought emerges. People who stop at thought are plagued with self-consciousness. They go through life trying to be aware of what they think, and how they think. In their thinking about thinking, what usually arises is the manifestation of lousy thinking and lots of dead-end alleys.

The Mindful Corporation points people to the place from which thought emerges, a place in which there is both a tremendous level of healing and an opportunity for lasting fulfillment. Why is this important in business? Larry Senn, CEO of Senn-Delaney Leadership, believes it's critical because, as he states, "There are enormous stresses and strains in organizations right now that lead to a lot of things, including churning people. One of the major issues on the mind of most leaders is retention. So, by nature, an organization in which people aren't frenzied and overly stressed will do a better job of holding onto talent."

So, how do we transport ourselves to a place where we can access this level of understanding? Unfortunately, the printed word can only get us to the threshold. Whether or not we step into the new room is up to each individual.

There is no one mechanism that we are aware of that works for everyone. We know the state and how to get to the threshold, but no one can say, "Do this, then we'll be there." Many consciously and intuitively know this is true. However, in our attempt to get there more regularly, we have convinced ourselves that we need to do something special. For some people, meditation works; for others, it's jogging. Some people require a crisis. The down side of crisis motivation is that those who need them to access a mindful place often codify crises as the only way that they can move into something new. They go from crisis to crisis, and end up living a life filled with difficulties. They are continually putting themselves in harm's way for good reason—to feel healthy. Now, that may sound peculiar, but let us provide an example. While working with the prisoners at the Hawaii State Prison, we asked the inmates why there seemed to be so many fights taking place. The answer was at first surprising. The prisoners had discovered, on a purely experiential level, that they couldn't be mind-filled and fight successfully. Like all successful athletes have found, they were at their best when they were in "the zone," what we call mindful, and the feelings one gets when in this place are euphoric. So, in the prisoners' minds, the thinking was that to fight was to feel euphoric. It makes no sense, but there is logic in it. This is the same kind of thinking and logic used by people who feel that crises are good. When we take a step back and look at the behavior, it makes no sense, but there is a logical reason for it. It takes a crisis for these people to access that free-flow state of mind through which all these wonderful thoughts or feelings come forward. We hope to make clear that we don't need crises to access a mindful state.

If, however, we persist in operating out of a mind-filled state where crisis is our only link to this flow mode we call mindfulness, then all we can expect in the long run is burnout. We worked with an executive who had been put into a brand new position for which he had no experience. He was the eldest executive on the team and he was surrounded by a group of hard-charging youthful peers. His boss was a "take no prisoners" type of guy. Our older executive couldn't see what he was doing; his mind was filled with anxiety and stress. The net effect was that his family was unhappy. He wasn't getting any sleep. He was aging prematurely. And about 90 percent of his decisions and actions were bad. At one point he said, "I don't know if I am being schizophrenic or paranoid." When asked if he knew what those terms meant, he admitted, "No." We told him that a schizophrenic individual is a person whose mind is filled with thoughts that are all believed. A paranoid individual is one whose mind is filled with thoughts, but the individual doesn't believe a single one.

We asked him what he thought the common dimension was. He immediately saw that he was bouncing back and forth between the two. In that lower state, not only was his mind filled with thoughts, but he was chasing all of them equally. Each had the same meaning for him and he was try-ing to act on all of them. It didn't take long before he'd lost the discerning mechanisms of wisdom and perspective.

The consequence of the mind-filled state is physical, emo-tional, and psychological burnout. And when people melt down they become difficult to get along with, non-commu-nicative, make poor choices, and change directions arbitrar-ily. There is no continuity or consistency to their actions. They are always in a state of fatigue. So they are doing things to battle the state and cope with the symptoms, which can include taking everything from caffeine to amphetamines. If they used to smoke cigarettes a little bit, they now smoke a lot. Every action is a counter to a symptom. And when that person then interacts with the organization from that state of mind, the effects cascade throughout the whole system.

The antidote to operating from a mind-filled state is to come from a place of emergent wisdom, as opposed to simply going deeper into the pain. If someone is locked in pain, the best thing for them to do is to give up on what they're doing because it's not working. Now that may seem like a strange bit of advice, but a client of ours once told us, "As long as the person you are coaching feels that he or she has the answer, you have a challenge in front of you. There is no willingness to listen." When in search of an answer, if we're stuck doing just more of what we've been doing, we tend to remain in search mode and that leads us only deeper into pain.

Coming From Wisdom

As humans, we are fascinating and extremely capable creatures. Frequently, we know that no matter how hard we grind away on a problem, we aren't going to get an answer. At that moment when the realization "I don't know" first arises, we are actually accessing a higher source. So our way from pain to emergent wisdom is, if we can't solve a problem within a few seconds, we let it go. Now that may seem like a terribly ambiguous answer. And we often initially hear, "That doesn't work for me." So let's follow that typical dialogue.

"Well, OK, explain why it doesn't work and let's see if we can put a different spin on it."

"I'll have a problem that I can't bring to resolution immediately; I try to keep it in the forefront and keep working at it."

"Describe that process to me."

"Well, I keep asking questions; I keep talking to people while I analyze and explore the problem. Only then do I come up with a solution."

"Describe the moment of solution. Is it after you do some amount of a specific activity that you know you are going to come to the solution?"

"No, it's never like that. I never know how much activity I need, or how much study, research, or analysis I have to do before I come up with a solution. Sometimes it happens sooner, sometimes it happens later."

"That's the very point. The mechanism you are talking about is relatively arbitrary. The next time you are hit with an issue, do what you feel you need to do, but become aware of the moment of solution. What I propose is that at the moment before you got the solution, you had forgotten the problem. It was out of mind. You either said, 'I don't know what is coming of this,' or you walked away from it, or you were in the shower, or it was just before you fell asleep. Regardless of the situation, the issue and the problem were not on your mind. You weren't actively, consciously going after the solution."

In 9 cases out of 10, the response is, "You are absolutely right. It was the moment when the problem was not a problem. It was the moment when I could surrender to the problem—the fact that I did not have a solution—and I could walk away from it. The solution then came to me when I was driving the car."

Going to that place of quiet is not easy, especially when the perceived and "normal" reality is to keep "at it" as diligently as possible. Again, the reason for this is that in business, the traditional definition of health is what is considered "normal." We are healthy if where we are is not uncomfortable. However, the level of discomfort we learn to put up with does not necessarily indicate that we are in a healthy space. Instead, it is our level of ease and gracefulness in how we approach our work that indicates health. As we get more comfortable with this understanding, it will appear to many that we are just lucky or it will not appear that we are "working hard enough," even though our results are in place.

The Changing Landscape

If accomplishing more with greater ease and no burnout sounds too good to be true, then it's time to take a different look at the way we're doing business. This becomes especially apparent when we look out over the constantly changing landscape of business where just as a new peak pushes its way up in front of us, the one we've been standing on crumbles away. Rather than adapting to these undulations as they are encountered, we're finding that the various business camps are becoming more rigid and entrenched, eschewing flexibility and fortifying their stands to deal with change.

There is the "swim with the sharks" camp, the "take no prisoners" camp, the "just feel" camp or the "just follow instructions" camp, the "no whining" camp, the "get on with it" camp, and on and on. These camps are continually defining themselves and stating more clearly why, "Our philosophy is the best philosophy." But as Bob Pratt, CEO of the Los Angeles Chapter of Volunteers of America, warns, "We can have great organizational theory here but if what we are doing isn't accomplishing anything, how good is that? What is the advantage of growth if you are just going to be growing more stuff that doesn't work or, scarier still, makes things worse?"

The unfortunate news is that the more rigidly we define the boundaries of our camps, the less likely we are to embrace any wisdom from another camp. There are a million and one philosophies out there, many that are very inflexibly defined and demand literal adherence. Unfortunately, such fundamentalism allows only limited growth or adaptation to the world as it changes. We hear from the adherents of these philosophies, "Here are the Ten Commandments of Business. If your company's holy books are not organized according to these Ten Commandments of Business, you're not only damned, you're doomed." Creating the Mindful Corporation is not about imposing difficult thoughts; it's about allowing our innate wisdom to emerge. Corporate fundamentalism enshrined by those "who know" leads to nothing but greater fundamentalism and little, if any, real understanding.

What we are calling corporate fundamentalism is nothing more than conventional wisdom enthroned. When we speak of conventional wisdom, we're describing understanding that comes from memory; from what we already know, have learned, or what we have previously experienced or thought. In the case of organizations, the source of this conventionality is what we call collective memory. We become very good at recalling how we did things previously. Unfortunately, when new and creative solutions are called for, all that collective memory can muster is a level of cleverness, a new rehashing of what has undoubtedly been repeated before.

Some may point to the fact that what they've done before has always worked. Unfortunately, past success does not take into account current conditions, and conditions today are very different from those just a few years ago.

In business, as in life, we invariably reach a point of pain or discomfort in any and every operation we encounter or undertake. At that moment, we have two choices. We can either go deeper into the pain, where we ultimately find we're creating more of the same, or we can enable a place of wisdom. From the former approach, we may find temporary relief. From a place of wisdom, as we will demonstrate throughout this book, what changes is our relationship to pain—our fears of it and our need to end it.

Business As We Tend To Know It

As society has evolved, we've become more aware, almost in spite of ourselves, but our wisdom has not kept up with our level of awareness. By being aware, we have become more conscious of the variables life throws at us. This is especially true in the world of business. However, without wisdom, the only thing we can focus on is the content of our awareness, not how we become aware. When we focus only on content, our minds become filled with the noise and minutia that keep us from the spaciousness required to look beyond the noise and clutter. On one level, we are becoming more sensitive. On another, we are not increasing our level of wisdom to handle the sensitivity.

The result is mind-filledness, instead of the mindfulness necessary to open us to greater wisdom. When we are mind-filled, unable to receive or access more of anything life presents us, we begin to see stress levels rise. We become more suspicious of others and their motives. We close ourselves off to the greater good in favor of me-first attitudes that rely on such things as "pay for performance" as the sole means of feeling any possible job satisfaction. What's the alternative? An ethic that gains its rewards from a greater inner satisfaction. Some may say that an inner satisfaction doesn't pay the bills. But that is a mind-filled perspective. We have become so accustomed to job dissatisfaction based on our outer reward systems that it has become business as usual. By coming from a source of inner satisfaction, we begin doing our job better because it feels better, with greater spirit, results, and higher performance—and that pays the bills.

So how does our work become so mind-filled? Not too surprisingly, our work becomes mind-filled when we lead mind-filled lives. In place of wisdom, we've developed conscious mind tricks like memorizing values, making to-do lists, focusing on external results, or reframing situations to help us make it through. Reframing allows us to re-picture events from a different perspective. Is reframing bad? No, but there are a number of failings inherent within it. First, we are still re-reframing the same dissatisfying event. Second, its effects are short-lived. And third, while seemingly a simple technique, it actually takes a great deal of effort to accomplish. For example, let's say we lost the involuntary ability to breathe and we had to consciously fill and empty our lungs with air. On one level, we could say, "It's good we can make this conscious choice because it helps us stay alive." On another level, it takes a lot of time, energy, concentration, and effort to consciously breathe each and every breath.

When we run out of time, energy, concentration, and effort, we say things like I need to get away, I need to change my life to a simpler life, or the price is not worth the reward. As stress levels increase, we make "me-first" statements, and take on "me-first" attitudes. Why? Because we don't have the energy to see beyond our mind-filled existence. Purely outer resources, like money and the trappings of life, motivate us. We feel more alienated. We begin noticing the differences between people rather than our connections. Taken to an extreme, we become either threatened or frightened by people and events, even with those who are the closest to us. And since we are not alone in this world, as more people find themselves in mind-filled states interacting with others in mind-filled states, we discover that what emerges out of those interactions is not wisdom but terribly cluttered thinking that only compounds the difficulties. By continuing this pattern, we create a complex, deeply woven matrix of unhealthy choices and possibilities. Bob Gunn, CEO of Gunn Partners, an international consulting firm, believes that, "People don't slow down enough to really ask themselves what is fundamental. There is so much emphasis on making something happen that it doesn't matter what is being done as long as people are busy and taking action."

International's® CEO John Horne would agree. As he says, "I find that people get their minds so cluttered they can't define their purpose. They fill their minds up with all this data coming at them, and they don't have a way of saying, 'What am I trying to do and what is relevant?' Then they don't have a way of getting rid of all the clutter because they don't know what they are trying to do with it."

In contrast to this way of thinking, if we make the assumption that there is an innate state of health, a wisdom available to all of us that we can tap into that operates involuntarily like our breathing, then we can literally breathe new life into our workplaces. The proof of its innate quality is evident when we become conscious of coming to the end of our rope. What do we see when people become conscious enough that they can take no more of their mind-filled existence? They start living their lives with inner and simpler rewards. What we have found is that we can go to that same simplified place at work without having to forsake everything we may already have.

Living Inside Out

The illusion we are operating under is that we get good feelings from the efforts we put into our work. But as long as those feelings are motivated by outer rewards, they don't last. The brain, being as sharp as it is, makes the conclusion, "The more effort I put into something, the more good feelings I get," and this assumption is exactly what leads us astray. What may seem counter-intuitive is that the good feelings do not come from effort or behavioral activities or results achieved. Those are all outside-in remunerations. Lasting reward comes from the good feelings we get from the inside out. These are feelings like inspiration, gratitude, connection, compassion, and humor that are not contingent on the outside world. If we can access the states of mind called inspiration or gratitude, then no matter where we look, we see things to be inspired by or grateful for. We aren't searching for things to be grateful for, but we are *in* the state of gratitude. And out of that state comes the ability to see things through grateful eyes.

Our approach in the past has been to think of all the things we are grateful for and that would supposedly create a healthy state. All it does, though, is create a very temporary good feeling, one that contains the seeds of stress because it takes effort to accomplish that feeling. The key point here is that healthier, high-performance states are available to us not when we get caught within the frenetic complexity of our operations, but once we relax.

We can try this for ourselves the next time we notice that life is a grind. We stop, let our thoughts pass through, and we find that we return to a more mindful state. We don't *go to it*, but *return to it.*

People who focus on the minutia stay in the bogged-down world of comprehension. People who step back and get a broader perspective of what is going on step up to a greater level of understanding. This is what Albert Einstein was talking about when he said, "The same level of thinking that caused our problems can't be used to solve them." The key is perspective.

The Surrounding Ambiguity

To see and understand this larger picture of the world of business we're describing requires relationships that are open to interaction and a willingness to listen with a sense of open-mindedness toward one other. This means that we see innocence in others rather than suspicion and fear. While we will discuss this idea in greater detail in Chapter 8, for now, seeing innocence means we see life in action, the obvious nature of thought, and are willing to accept the ambiguity that exists around us. Our managers have been trained to trained to think that ambiguity is a bad thing, and a great deal of our quantification-based business education has been directed toward sanitizing it out.

Accepting ambiguity is being comfortable in a state of not knowing. In that state, we can either drive ourselves to make things up or we can be open to our intuition and understanding. In business, the idea of living our lives in a state of not knowing is terrifying. This is especially true when Wall Street's quarterly reports, by law, seek to make everything crystal clear to an investor.

What we miss when we want to make the waters less murky too quickly, however, is the often profound nature of real innovation. When we are uncomfortable in a state of not knowing, we often latch onto the first answer that pops up as a way to relieve our fears and discomfort. As Gunn Partners' CEO Bob Gunn makes clear, "Just because a thought pops into someone's head, doesn't mean they have to act upon it or pay attention to it." The nature of interactions, however, is such that if we allow that first answer to further interact with other possibilities, what then emerges may have been absolutely inconceivable previously. That is what we call wisdom. What we have found is that our resistance to ambiguity is equal to our resistance to humility—our willingness to not know the answer—and that greater answers are available to us if we wait quietly and respectfully. And in a manner that may seem counter-intuitive, by allowing ourselves to rest in a state of humility, what emerges might completely change our world.

A dramatic change such as this can happen because wisdom is actually a transcendent function. That does not mean that we hear angels sing whenever a moment like this takes place. Transcendent means to rise above. When we experience a true insight, we're having what might be called a moment of novel transcendence. The elevated wisdom that arises and the attendant vision that comes from this higher ground provide a perspective that allows us the potential to adjust our position and move forward to our new emergent understanding—a new level of thinking, as Einstein would describe it. The opposite of emergent wisdom is memory, which only gives us more of the same thinking.

What keeps us from realizing the potential of emergent wisdom and its novel transcendence is our mind-filled thinking and its source—memory.

Mind-filled Thinking

Mind-filled thinking is previous thought, re-thought. Imagine a person walking around carrying a palm computer wherever he or she goes. When life throws that person a curve, his or her habitual response is to go through their mental palm computer to see if he or she has had to deal with that curve or something similar before. It is like walking through life backwards, or driving a car forward, but by looking in the rearview mirror. With mind-filled thinking there is no room or time for the consideration of anything different because the mind is filled with conditioned or remembered responses, or an established idea of the way things are.

Where once we might have been able to tolerate mind-filled thinking in our organizations, today elements like pace and demand are making things less forgiving. Unfortunately, our mind-filled thinking, in turn, creates demanding and less-forgiving corporate cultures. It appears that with more to do, our margins become smaller. During the Industrial Age times, our margins for operating were wider. We felt we could give people the benefit of the doubt, and more time to come up with new solutions. But as we start to speed up and work under the illusion that we have less space to work in, the tolerances become more finite, and it takes on the look of being less forgiving for "all the right reasons." We have no room for error and no space for emergent ideas.

What we see are people performing under tremendous pressure. And those people, whose stress levels are rising, are also feeling unappreciated. The mind-filled thinker looks at this, and anger is not far behind. What they are failing to see is that their state of mind is at the root of their stress and their lack of appreciation. Feeling pressure and needing appreciation from the outside are the same state of mind, just focused on different topics.

What can be done for someone in this condition? Giving them what they want will only satisfy their short-term needs. The best and only long-term action that will work is for them to access a healthier mindful state as opposed to responding to a requested behavior. Mind-filled thinking keeps us from feeling our pressure or seeing our lack of appreciation in any other light than from a stressful, unappreciated state.

The answer is to get away from the content of our thinking and take a look at the quality of our thinking itself. Instead of asking why we are worried, which leads us back into the content of our thinking, we need to see *that* we are thinking. Once we get that perspective, we can move off the place on which we are stuck.

When we begin to look at the function of thought—not its content but the dynamics of thought—we find that it is nothing more than the manifestation of a formless state. The problem is that as soon as we recognize thought, we take one step away from the formlessness from which it emanated. Spaciousness is a step toward that source. The mindful state allows us to put some separation between our thoughts so that we can begin to see how our minds are cluttered with a million different things. When the mind is spacious, we can get clarity because we have created some breathing room with fewer things in the way to defuse the issue.

Spaciousness enables us to access the full range of the mind's capacities. The more spacious our minds, the greater access we have to wisdom, joy, and compassion, as well as memory and analysis.

Mind-filled Behaviors

Rather than allow spaciousness to occur, our mind-filled solutions turn toward more unhealthy kinds of distractions to get away from our discomfort. When the pain is truly great, the distraction can become even more severe, and takes the form of anything from abusive behavior of oneself and others, to drug and alcohol abuse or violence.

In the workplace, we see people all the time who are in pain or in unhealthy places and don't want to face their discomfort. They are often cruel to one another and find any number of alcohol or drug-induced avenues for escape. An unhealthy person is frequently a master of self-sabotage as well as capable of sabotaging the projects of others. Other manifestations include repeatedly not being present in conversations, calling in sick, stealing from the organization, or feeling the organization owes him.

However, all distractions are not as dramatic as those we have just mentioned. Because we have become accustomed to a certain level of distraction in our lives, we have come to accept a "normal" level of tension and stress. Our belief that some stress is good for us and that we "need" some pressure, threat, or insecurity to get things done is an example of this. For some, the way they prove their worth is to work to the point of fatigue; that is, "work hard, play hard." Our lives are full of slogans justifying this mind-filled existence..."No pain, no gain," "What goes up must come down," "The only fair measure of effort is results."

We have all seen tremendously capable people who seem to always screw up. They rarely do enough to sink the ship, but they can make it stall or list to one side. All we can do is scratch our heads and wonder why they do it. We also work with people who seem to have an uncanny *in*ability to solve problems effectively. At least it seems uncanny to those who can solve problems easily. One reason we get stuck in this unhealthy behavior is that we take what is normal for us as reality. When we're not in a state of mindfulness, we don't realize that our "normal" is something that we have conjured up ourselves. The mindful state begins the journey toward health. From that state comes the realization that our "normal" is of our own making. Over the course of years, we have received our kudos in business and in life by demonstrating how much stress and tension we can put up with and still look functional. We then perceive this stressed feeling as normal behavior. In actuality, all we have done is move our "normal" away from health.

The "normals" of the people who have a difficult time accessing their capabilities are so far removed from their healthy state that they can no longer see what health is. They can't access their *true* normal state. Their distracting thoughts, which are predominantly historical and based in memory, keep them locked in this conjured realm. This is why their solutions to problems all tend to look alike.

As the saying goes, "When your only tool is a hammer, every problem looks like a nail." What we want to do is provide the key to the tool cabinet so that we can access unlimited possible solutions to address all situations. When we come from a place of health, that is not only possible, it is normal and natural.

Chapter Two

Organizational Healthy Functioning

"The answer to today's business and personal challenges does not lie in harder or more frantic effort. We believe it lies in creating an organization in which things happen with greater ease, one with more collaboration instead of turf, and wiser, more thoughtful, decisions."

—

Larry E. Senn and John R. Childress

Ideals are fine when we are discussing the philosophical understanding of justice and equality, but idealized business practices rarely, if ever, find the light of day. The Mindful Corporation is not an ideal. It is a pragmatic and conscious enactment of how a real organization can re-create itself to thrive in a complex and ever-changing environment. So, what does it look like?

The Motivating Factor

On the surface, one might be hard-pressed to distinguish it from any other business. There are people performing tasks and getting the business of the day completed. The differences become more apparent as we delve deeper into how that daily business process takes place. What motivates those within a Mindful Corporation is very different from what motivates most corporate employees. First of all, the whole idea of motivation gets turned around. In most companies, human resource departments and senior management are continually involved in providing external enticements that will motivate work: raises, compensation and benefit packages, incentive allotments, rewards and acknowledgement ceremonies, and even the occasional motivational speaker. All of these factors share one common ingredient: They come from the outside as a way to instill an inner motivation.

While all of these elements are welcome, they are not a lasting means for creating motivated workers. Not only are these effects temporary, but, as time goes on, they require more and better benefits and continually greater incentives. Without an understanding of the source of motivation, we create systems that do nothing but reinforce its need. Let's take an extreme example to better explain this. Some of us use alcohol as a means of getting away from the pain of thinking. But the alcohol actually keeps us locked at the level of consciousness that causes us to need it. It is the same with motivation that comes from the outside in. Motivation without understanding and awareness of its source simply reinforces the level of consciousness that wants and needs motivation. The result is a vicious and repetitive cycle. We become addicted to the need as a way of keeping us going; as a way of coping. When we don't receive what we want from the outside, we begin questioning ourselves as to whether or not what we are doing is worth the effort. Because we see our environment, situation, and others as the source of our fulfillment, we will blame them when we don't feel healthy. We become victims of our circumstances. We seek out other methods to ease the discomfort caused by that lack of outer motivation. In those cases when external factors don't satisfy our need, our dissatisfaction is played out on the job. Quarrels and disagreements are "normal," and dysfunction is the acceptable practice for getting through the day.

From a positive perspective, when we find ourselves needing outside motivation, and we receive it, we are temporarily distracted from the thinking that creates the need that, in turn, allows us to see other possibilities and levels of consciousness. This includes exploring the possibility that there is another form of living other than the one that we are experiencing right now. We found this to be true when we were working in the Hawaii State Prison. Before we could get the inmates to entertain new thoughts, we had to encounter them immediately after they satisfied their distracting thoughts. It was almost counter-intuitive to the way in which they were being treated. We wanted to talk to the inmates the moment after they had a fight. We wanted to talk to them the moment they started to sober up. They were no longer filled by the same feelings and thinking that had pushed them toward acting out and from which they had wanted to be distracted. We didn't want to wait for days, because over that time, their old style of thinking would start to re-root, and the same habitual forms of distraction that made sense to them before were once again viable answers. By doing so, they could see the distraction for what it was…their thinking.

In the workplace, we might see this opportunity for another way of living taking place around reward and appreciation ceremonies. In an organization that doesn't understand this process, a reward and appreciation ceremony might be the final item on an agenda, offering a way of celebrating with everyone leaving on a high. Unfortunately, that feeling quickly falls away and people find themselves craving something more. An alternative approach we use in our meetings is to begin with rewards and appreciation and then go right into more perspective-building activities in which we focus and reflect on our thinking. This might be done through directed questions pointing toward our perceptions of appreciation or gratitude or even the work before us. This takes advantage of that moment we start to fall off the high, because that is where the opening for real teaching can take place, while we are feeling good inside and not distracted by our habitual ways of thinking.

In essence, we are saying that outside-in motivation is a way of distracting our thinking, thus providing temporary encouragement. However, when our motivation comes from within, we find that life's events are not seen as distractions, but merely as life's events. Our lives no longer require constant maintenance, encouragement, and effort because it comes from the inside out. In the mindful organization, motivation is one of the indicators of our momentary health. It's not the end product that recognizes good performance; it is the beginning step toward greater learning and deeper personal commitment. As Atmos Energy CEO Bob Best explains, "I always tell employees, 'there is no joy in making money. The joy is setting goals and accomplishing those goals. Whatever service you are providing is where you get your joy.'"

Mindfulness Begins at the Top

The recognition that mindfulness begins with the leaders of the organization is of paramount importance to success in the creation of the Mindful Corporation. The leader's job is to run the company; to have the vision that creates and sustains the philosophy out of which the organization—its leadership, individuals, and teams—operates. The mindful leader is quite different from the stereotypical boss. One immediately feels a stabilizing effect as opposed to a frenetic one around this person. It is not necessarily based on what this person knows at the moment, but rather the high degree of rapport we feel with him or her. In contrast, the mind-filled leader is always listening for content and trying to figure things out via that content. After a meeting with a leader like this, one feels exhausted and self-conscious. The frenzy itself is mind-boggling, and everything said is often challenged and must be fully supported. One continually feels on guard, searching for survival clues to get through the encounter. The alternative approach is found in the leader who listens not only for the content, but for something deeper; the grains of truth in what is being said and the feeling behind it. This does not mean that the content is unimportant, but the mindful leader is also listening for something different. And very quickly, so too, is the person he or she might be meeting with.

We walk into the room with a mindful leader and we feel a little nervous, but within a relatively short time we feel ourselves calming down. We feel listened to, and an interesting occurrence takes place. We find *ourselves* listening more completely. Not only are we listening for content, but for feelings and concepts as well. Thoughts and ideas pop into our heads that come from what is being said, but not *because* of what is being said. Without any conscious effort, our creativity kicks into gear. The questions that pop into our minds are different, deeper, furthering, rather than defensive. Ron Adams, former President of CNG Regulated Businesses, believes that "Everybody deserves great leadership. They deserve a safe work environment, both physically and emotionally, where they can deal with real issues and be themselves without fear of retribution. That then creates exceptional results."

When we walk into the office of a mind-filled leader, we immediately feel under the gun, scrutinized. In the worse case, we feel like we're constantly being tested. We leave feeling more nervous than when we walked in, more insecure, and not sure if anything positive could come out of that encounter.

Why is this true? With the mindful leader, there is perspective that comes from pause, from knowing and understanding quiet, from an appetite for really listening. With the mind-filled leader, there is little or no perspective. It is just a flow of old thoughts without any reflection. It's all reaction to content without any awareness or curiosity of what lies behind the ideas.

This is not a conscious action on the part of either leader. For the mind-filled leader, this way of acting is all his or her mind will allow. There's simply no space for any other way of being. For the mindful leader, the process is more intuitive; less reactionary. The key is listening to one's own inner voice, something we all do all day long as we go about our daily process of thinking and responding. Some of us are more aware of this ongoing inner dialogue than others, but it nonetheless exists for each of us and takes on a variety of tones and attitudes. The mindful leader, feeling comfortable in this intuitive state and aware of his or her thinking habits and patterns, can listen for an appropriate voice from within, other than the one that only offers criticism or analysis. In a similar instance, the mind-filled leader is more likely to be unaware that he or she is projecting his or her own insecurity—his or her fear of not knowing or having the right answer—onto a situation. By allowing more space, the mindful leader becomes more aware of his or her projections or more likely to recognize when they are projecting, and can allow an interaction to take place from a less personal and imposing perspective.

Within the Mindful Corporation, communication is not simply talking, giving feedback and exchange. There's a mutual dialoguing that takes place. There's not a lot of, "OK, I am going to give you feedback now." It is more like an ongoing conversation. The healthier the culture and the more responsive the organization, the more we find people who are talking with one another on an ongoing basis. Healthy relationships are all about ongoing dialogue. This is not just an exchange of data and information, but a willingness and openness for dialogue.

We're not talking about action team discussions, brainstorming, green light discussions, or re-engineering company processes. All of these can be useful when used appropriately. Dialogue is a means of stimulating original thought with less mental activity. Business consultants like Peter Senge have pointed out that in discussion, views are presented, debated, defended, and compared. In dialogue, issues are explored, new views are discovered, common ground is identified, assumptions are suspended, and there is no personal investment in the outcome.

This is not simply a semantic difference, but one of intent as well. Dialogues are about inquiry and learning, about considering thoughts and reflection, or discovering shared visions. They are an attempt to discover common meaning, to hear and understand many different perspectives that allow the synthesis of a whole system view. It provides an opportunity to question our assumptions and beliefs and to explore what it means to think collectively.

Discussion is about telling, fixing, selling ideas, or persuading. It is intended to gain agreement or deliver a vision, to advocate a single perspective, and bring individuals into conformance with the group. It's about solving problems, not exploring new ideas. So consequently, discussion is about parts, not wholes, and finding what some may think is the "best" solution, but not necessarily a new solution.

Dialogues start from and create greater respect and rapport, and, therefore, more trust develops between participants and within the group. When we are able to remove our personal investment in the outcome—finding a solution we can take credit for—we open up to learning as a core competency. And by creating this true collegial relationship, we prepare the group for truly creative and original thinking because no one is trying to outdo or outshine anyone else.

Dialogue, in the fashion we're describing, requires an ability to suspend our assumptions and beliefs and to let go of our prejudices and preconceived notions—our "favorite" views. This may seem like an impossible task within any group of people, but when everyone is aligned around the desire to explore and discover new possibilities, and not attached, via ego, to the outcome, remarkable ideas emerge.

What impedes this process of dialogue is our impatience—our need to speed up, or stated differently, our unwillingness to slow down. This mind-filled state might come about because we are trying to fit this event into our hectic schedule, rather than providing the appropriate time and space needed. What also restricts our dialogue from realizing all the available possibilities are our preconceived notions of what we think this process should look like and what we think the outcome should be. We often get stuck here because we are invested in the outcome.

Now to some, the deconstructing of a meeting like this might seem an invitation to chaos. But by using a facilitator who is not attached to the outcome, we keep everyone on track and on task. In addition, by setting a time limit for the dialogue, we can provide some structure. So why is this process healthier?

In an environment in which feedback, as opposed to dialogue, is emphasized, people often become very self-conscious about their behaviors, putting a tremendous amount of energy into changing something that they don't do all the time. For example, suppose we're attending a presentation and one of the presenters is having a bad day, delivering his portion of the presentation poorly. Someone might give him feedback on how to improve his performance, without an understanding that everybody has good days and bad days. Wanting to act on the feedback, he then spends time and energy making adjustments to behavior that was initiated because he was simply feeling poorly or "off."

When we can stay in dialogue, the conversation doesn't just occur when something doesn't work, but on a regular basis. A co-worker is going through a difficult period. He asks, "Have you noticed that I have been off?" The dialogue is simply, "It appears to me that you haven't been the normal, bubbly person...." He responds, "Help me out, here." This is opposed to: "Listen, Fred, why don't you sit down, I have some feedback I want to give you." In dialogue, there is a mutuality and an availability to our interactions at the same time we are ready to hear it and make a difference.

Communicating Beyond Sharing Information

Dialoguing is one aspect of the Mindful Corporation's communication approach. Within the overall scheme, people communicate openly and freely. They are aware of content, as well as tone, while building rapport. They listen both with humility and a desire to be influenced, without losing their perspective or position. That doesn't happen when we are content-driven because all content is delivered from a similar level of perspective. This is why tone and rapport need to be equal partners in this process. Becoming conscious of the feeling behind the content is essential in communication, as is the level of comfort people feel toward each other. If we feel openly received, we're much more likely to respond in kind. We have been in meetings where one group sits on one side of the room and another on the other side awaiting the arrival of the director. No one says anything across the established lines of the groupings. When the director arrives and seats himself, he pronounces, "So, we begin." And the meeting is launched with great mistrust and little real communication. Americans in Japan often find themselves feeling incredibly impatient as their Japanese counterparts discuss seemingly frivolous things with them about family, sports, and the like. The last five minutes of the meeting address "the business." Yet, once rapport has been established, that's all that is sometimes required.

Communication in a Mindful Corporation is also based on listening and being able to tap into our own quiet places where the mind slows down. From this perspective, we can listen from the highest form of listening—open to be influenced by any possibility and respectfully curious. There is a subtle distinction to be made here. We don't want to go into an interaction *thinking*, "I want to be influenced." If we do, we lose the wisdom that enables us to differentiate between what works and what doesn't. If, however, we enter an interaction with the state of mind that "I am truly open to being influenced," we can gain many grains of truth from the person with whom we are speaking and listening. In doing so, we still have the capability to perceive when "that was off base." This ability doesn't come from listening solely to the content spoken, but from perspective. In the mind-filled organization, we often encounter people who either refuse to listen or listen very selectively. They're blind to the filters of their thinking and deal primarily with information, rarely going out of their way to assist others or be influenced by what they hear.

Judgment to Block

One way we keep ourselves from being influenced is through judgment. In this instance, people who are driven by judgment often use their own thoughts as a filter, so that what is being said to them needs to make it through the filter of their thinking in order for them to hear it. For example, if Ruth were to profess a particular problem with Elizabeth because her point of view was different than Elizabeth's, whatever idea Elizabeth might put forward would be seen through the filter of Ruth's judgment. As might be expected, the more judgmental a person is, the finer the filter's screen, so very little gets through. It can get to the point where the person who is really judgmental no longer comes from "Should I be influenced?" but their stance is "I do the influencing."

Now, there are those who will say, "But I have to be able to get this information out. The content is important." What we have found is that no matter what we try to do, the content will always come through. The key is to make the content the background of these interactions, not the foreground. That may seem like a radical perspective, but when all parties come from this direction, real dialogue takes place without the attendant stresses, political undercurrents, and dysfunctions.

A State of Everlasting Becoming

It is important to emphasize that the Mindful Corporation is not striving for some profound perfection as an end state. Rather, it realizes that the process is a journey. The driving insight behind this thinking is that we are always in relationship. What does that mean? From the interaction of quarks at the subatomic particle level to the interaction of galactic forces in the universe, whatever the scale or time frame, everything is ultimately in relation to everything else. If we take this stance with our personal relationships, that we are always together, something very interesting emerges—a greater gentleness—that we are in process, a process Plato called "everlasting becoming." The more short-term we see our relationships, the more we feel we need to get it right in a short period of time and the less forgiving we are. Take, for instance, the example of a divorced couple who share the raising of their children. They are in a relationship whether they are married or not. What usually happens in these circumstances, with those who are successful at it, is that they learn to be gentle with one another. They tend to let go of a lot of the communication problems that they had in the past that were often content-driven. Once the content loses its power, they can start to communicate with each other again. This is why we often hear people in this situation say, "We're better friends now than when we were married."

These people realize that, because of the kids, they are always going to be in a relationship. It is just not the form they originally thought it would be, and their communication improves measurably. The same is true in organizations that have a long-term perspective and therefore communicate with each other more gently. Direct evidence of this is that these organizations often have very supportive alumnae. This is a mindset toward communication created within the organization, but flowing as part of the culture, which, as we have found in our work, comes directly from leadership.

The Consequence of Good Communication is Excellent Teamwork

As in any healthy organization, teamwork is of paramount importance. In the traditional sense of the word, teamwork takes on a variety of forms depending on the need of the moment. Sometimes it looks like collaboration, and other times it is singularly led or with collaboration showing up later. The key here is that the mechanism driving how anything gets done is determined by the wisdom of the moment and not by any proscriptive behavior. The external variables are urgency, time, buy-in, and the nature of the challenge or job.

We see this played out in situations in which a team may work together in a brainstorming session. They might then split up responsibilities and do different parts of the job and bring the completed effort back for consensus. We might also see one person take the lead on a project and direct the group. All of this is determined by situation. Organizations that do this with ease create what we call "high-performance" teams, capable of producing their best work, whether individually or collectively.

It is important to understand that in trying to re-create a high-performance state and teach others its ins and outs, business professionals and consultants have taken what looked like disparate behaviors and taught them very linearly. They looked at teamwork, accountability, communication, coaching, and strategy and taught them as separate pieces. Then they said, "Oh, by the way, they are all linked, even though we are teaching them as separate pieces."

In the Mindful Corporation, we realize that the separateness of these issues is totally an illusion. There is no difference between teamwork and accountability, teamwork and communication, or teamwork and leadership. They are all manifestations of our ability to be in the moment.

From this perspective, the process of coaching takes on a

very different cast as well. In a mindful organization, coaching is 90 percent listening and 10 percent talking. Its focus is on performance, humility, and rapport. It's not an activity solely driven by performance—corrective or preventative—but is a normal, conversational dimension of the organization's culture and values. In other words, it's dialogue. It is educational as well as transforming. Let us provide an example. As an executive, I'm working on a project and I'm starting to feel frustrated in not being able to push it through quickly enough. I feel this is something on which we need to move ahead, but the actualization process within the organization is slow at best. I come to a colleague and say, "I just don't know what to do about this." And the dialogue begins.

Within the context of that dialogue, my colleague is listening to what I'm saying, asking a question or two to clarify my thinking, but mostly he is listening to me. In my description of the issues, suddenly a new possibility pops into my mind. It was something that had not previously occurred to me, and it catches me a bit by surprise. My colleague smiles and says simply, "I think that is it. Why don't you go try it?"

How did my colleague "coach" me? As mentioned earlier, the essence of successful coaching in this mindful approach is that 90 percent of the process is listening and 10 percent is talking. In addition, 90 percent of that 10 percent spent on talking is merely asking questions, and the remaining 10 percent of the 10 percent is actually making statements.

We saw this at work with the management board of British Telecom (BT). They came into their session very distracted about how they don't come together enough to talk about strategy. So, the first day we were together all we did was touch on a few things and intervene only when the dialogue was going sidewise. For the most part on that first day, they just had to get past their distracting thoughts. At the end of the first day, we presented a few ideas about forgiveness and what we call "the vertical dimension of understanding": how our state of consciousness rises and falls along a continuum from anger and mistrust to generosity and forgiveness.

The next day they came in and said, "It was really important what we talked about in terms of strategy, but for my team, I want more about forgiveness. We need to learn more about the vertical dimension of understanding. That's what I want my team to walk away with."

The point we then made with them was that they couldn't have heard what little we presented as deeply as they did if they had remained stuck in their distractions. There is an inverse relationship between distraction and our depth of listening. For coaches this means that we are not only mindful of those who seek our coaching, but we must be aware of our own distractions in order to be there for those we coach. It is our belief that the whole focus of coaching, teamwork, accountability, and facilitation is for the leader or coach to create what we call the learnable moment.

It is important to understand that the learnable moment does not necessarily come when we are taught something. When our distractions fall away, we are open to possibilities and our innate wisdom can rise up. That moment of personal insight immediately changes what we have habitually believed or previously thought. It is an immediate emptying of the filled mind and an awareness of what is possible when we live mindfully.

Vertical Dimension of Understanding

- Wise, Inspired
- Grateful, Generous, Forgiving
- Creative, Innovative
- Resourceful
- Hopeful, Optimistic
- Appreciative, Compassionate
- Patient, Understanding
- Sense of Humor
- Flexible, Adaptive, Cooperative
- Curious, Interested
- Impatient, Frustrated
- Irritated, Bothered
- Worried, Anxious
- Defensive, Insecure
- Judgmental, Blaming
- Self-Righteous
- Stressed, Burned-Out
- Mistrustful
- Angry

© 2000 SENN-DELANEY LEADERSHIP

How does an organization deal with someone who is reluctant to be open to the learnable moment? Once we take into account that occasionally everyone's performance slips, we need to address a person's willingness to improve, change, and be coached. The slope of improvement then needs to meet the parameters of required performance. If coaching is part of the normal fabric of the company and is not seen as punitive or episodic, then improvement is a viable measure of performance. If someone is not willing to engage in that process, then they are not performing his or her job. But if change and coaching are seen as either punitive or episodic, then performance is driven by insecurity, and that insecurity needs to be addressed as much as the performance itself.

We have found that for the most part, 99 percent of the people in the world are willing to dialogue and engage in this process. Even people who are extremely shy or introverted will talk to someone. The issue is not the activity of dialoging, but the thinking we harbor with the person with whom we interact. Reluctance to participate normally connotes a perceived threat. If we approach these people from a mindful perspective, they will eventually shed their reluctance and join in. Often, with those who are reluctant, this is the *only* way they will join in.

A Healthy Role for Policy and Procedures

Policies and procedures are only effective when they provide clarity, wisdom, and a source of alignment to make things easier. If they don't, they should be re-examined and changed. The ultimate objective of policy and procedure is not strict compliance, but understanding. This is not a list of dos and don'ts. But this is rarely the case in a mind-filled organization. When our policies and procedures sound like the "word of the Lord," they make little sense to people.

We have found that rules and procedures come into existence to support our models for doing business. They are meant to represent our "best thinking" at the moment. When the model changes, or the quality of our thinking improves, the rules and procedures have to change, too. It is for this reason that they should always come after the fact. When rules and procedures precede the model and no longer point toward the healthy state from which those thoughts emerge, a stifling bureaucracy sets in, and there is little or no room left for growth or change.

For example, our company has a hard time getting our consultants to fill out a certain set of documentation papers on time and on a regular basis. There are excellent reasons for the documentation and an equal amount of reasons why it is essential to our operations. When the documentation was initially introduced, rules and procedures were created to establish a model for behavior about the completion of this form. And the company has had nothing but difficulties with the administration of this documentation ever since.

We would probably have been better served if we had found out first what worked before the model for receiving this documentation was established. Instead, the system and its attendant behaviors were made mandatory. Hindsight has suggested that perhaps we could have examined the criteria behind the documentation and been willing to redesign it after the fact. We could then acquire all the necessary information, but not necessarily via the same documentation procedures with which people, despite the best efforts of a gently cajoling staff, still seem to have so much difficulty.

The problem is that once a procedure becomes sacrosanct and surrounded by a system to implement it, it is rarely questioned. This area of rules and procedures points out a valuable process within the Mindful Corporation—the willingness to question what is held sacrosanct by the organization. This questioning process is not always as easy as it may sound. Companies tend to hold on to the way things have always been done for very good reasons, in spite of the fact that there may be better ways. This is also true of individuals who hold onto rules or procedures for very good reasons as well. Within the Mindful Corporation, there is an awareness of the attachments we tend to make, but also an understanding that these, too, are rooted in thought. By being open to where we get stuck in our thinking, we can make sure that what we are holding sacred in our organizations is worthwhile. A corporation with the courage to discard what is no longer needed is constantly making room for the new.

The Power of Relating

As mentioned previously, the real solution to making all of this work in the Mindful Corporation is our willingness to relate. When we see our relationships with others as ongoing and long-term, we establish a gentleness over time that allows and ameliorates our working together with ease. In many cases, these relationships flourish well beyond the scope of the organization and continue regardless of employment. These bonds also form the foundation for future alliances and partnerships. The reason for this is that successful employees in a Mindful Corporation are willing to access their wisdom, mutual respect, and innate sense of health. This is at the heart of all decisions and actions that are made. We see this in long-term relationships where people understand that form—how relationships are formalized, and the daily details of life associated with that formalization—is not as significant or powerful as living in the presence of integrity and health.

If we understand that values are limitless, that they don't stop at the boundaries of the organization, then relationships based on those values continue as well. But many mind-filled organizations are intent on building boundaries to protect proprietary information, and a tremendous amount of time, energy, and resources are put into defending intellectual capital products. When someone leaves an organization, his friends within those old organizations are often restrained and discouraged by rules and regulations from continuing the dialogue and the relationship with their former colleague. What would happen if, instead of limiting that extended contact, we encouraged and supported alumnae in furthering the message of the organization wherever they might travel. When we view relationships as long-term, then we do whatever we can to enable each other to be as successful as possible in any new endeavor.

The problem, of course, is proprietary information. We waste a tremendous amount of money and effort worrying about who is going to steal our ideas and instituting procedures to protect them, rather than thinking, how can we get these ideas out to the public so they can produce even greater good? Part of the fear that keeps us guarding what we perceive as proprietary is first that these ideas are ours, and second that we are not going to have another good idea.

Goethe once said, "No one can take from us the joy of first becoming aware of something, the so-called discovery. But if we also demand the honor, it can be utterly spoiled for us, for we are usually not the first. What does discovery mean, and who can say that he has discovered this or that? After all it's pure idiocy to brag about priority, for it's simply unconscious conceit, not to admit frankly that one is a plagiarist."

What we have found is that the more open we are with ideas, the more often deeper ideas arise. When we start protecting our ideas, and living under the fear of this proprietary nature, we greatly limit the possibilities. This is an excellent indication of an organization's willingness and/or difficulty in changing. The degree to which we see the dynamic, living nature of ideas is the degree to which the evolution of an organization becomes more graceful. Organizations that tend to evolve over time, and maintain their timeliness, are not wedded to yesterday's thoughts. Or as Bob Gunn puts it, "We are sowing the seeds of our own limitations the more we stay wedded to the ideas of the past."

3M is an excellent example of an organization that has moved on from the ideas upon which it was founded, and has succeeded on the strength of its new innovations. The open culture they have created was built for innovation and greatly enhanced the scope and scale of its business. In contrast, Apple Computers lost a good deal of market share through its decision early on in its development to make proprietary and protect its operating platforms. IBM, which has continued to dominate the computer business, spread PC use to the world by opening up its systems and pushing new ideas. To Apple's credit, it has never been averse to trying something new and different, but what might it have become if it had made its platforms more accessible and less proprietary?

To be willing to let go of yesterday's thoughts requires an organization that is willing to provide a safe place for taking risks. At one level of understanding within the Mindful Corporation, the notion of risk does not exist. Now, without getting tied to some mystical misunderstanding here, in a mindful environment, what needs to be done is obvious. There is no risk in taking a step forward that is obvious. Failure is a relative term, based on our concept of success. But what we find is that it is easily offset by support, humility, and a willingness to stay engaged within the organization.

To the untrained eye, risk, courage, and commitment are scary words. However, when we come from a state of wisdom and inspiration, open to the possible and all its configurations, the choices we make seem obvious. They don't appear risky or as if we have to summon courage in order to make them. We may realize the leap taken after the fact when someone says, "Boy, that was a courageous thing to do." But the only way that observer can make a point of courageousness is to inject a sense of his or her own insecurity. Risk can only exist in insecurity.

Psychological vulnerability is another related idea. Being vulnerable is also a very outside-in way of perceiving one's place in the world. Vulnerability is allowing someone else to do something to us. We speak about being vulnerable to attack. When we open our feelings to others, we make ourselves vulnerable to their response. People get into a habit of "doing" vulnerability or "doing" risk-taking. We often see this played out by the person in an organization who prides him- or herself on being the black sheep. This is often a person who is purposefully on the outside taking the opposite direction of the organization. Any organizational route is seen as limiting or is mistrusted, but whatever the reason given, the black sheep always maintains an outside-in perspective. The key to turning this behavior inside out is to see where it is coming from—our willingness to live in a place of our own projected insecurity. When we understand how our thinking creates such things as vulnerability, we can begin taking greater accountability for our actions in the world, and such things as taking risks become nothing more than simply living life.

Measuring and Evaluating—The Quantification Factor

One reason business has tried to limit the scope of relationships is that it is so difficult to measure. But if just doing the job is no longer what we are solely accountable for, how do we go about measuring and evaluating our people? Within the structure of a mind-filled work environment, it is "normal" for people to feel that their results provide a sense of fulfillment for them. Results are something tangible, existing outside, which can be held up and pointed to with pride. From this state, we are seeing the world from an outside-in perspective. Our outside results make us feel better about ourselves inside. Consequently, when we base our feeling of job satisfaction on these outer measures, it invariably leads to frustration, lack of fulfillment, and stress. The feeling derived is too short-lived. Soon, we have to deliver more and better results, or something gets in our way while trying to produce them that causes stress and frustration with the system. We discover, time and again, that this outside-in perspective provides little lasting job satisfaction and is actually a very unhealthy level of awareness. In the long term, this results-oriented thinking creates a driven organization that is often earmarked by short-term results, arrogance, insecurity, self-esteem issues, dirty politics, superficial fixes to problems, and an inordinate amount of stress and tension.

From the mindful perspective, we see that individuals who are capable of honestly seeing their results as a manifestation of their own state of fulfillment are much better off at the end of the day. They have the capacity to maintain their bearings and their balance, as well as continue to grow and enhance themselves and their company. They move with change relatively easily, and respond to issues and challenges in an appropriate fashion. Within this structure, then, people are evaluated not only on getting results, but on such things as their ability to change, their response to new issues and challenges, and their support of their fellow employees. As Atmos Energy's Bob Best explains, "An organization's health operates from inside-out no differently than a person's does." In spite of this, our measurement capabilities often fail to take this into account.

Ron Adams, one of Bob Best's protégés, continues this thinking by adding, "In fact, one measure of a healthy organization should be how wisdom is shared."

Often the reason for not addressing these more intangible measures is because it is simply easier to measure output. But what we can see in those environments that drive this particular measure is a plentitude of negative behaviors: absenteeism, personal and public sabotage, poor working relationships, and lots of stress-related illnesses. For an organization focused solely on results, this is the price that business has to pay. If, however, the focus were on the health of the organization and the people within it, getting tangible results would be just part of the tapestry that makes up the way we work.

Now there will be some who say, "But we're in business to get results and be profitable." They are absolutely right. Performance, values representation, and strategic determination are integral and imperative parts of the business process. But how those issues are driven is the critical factor. What we are suggesting is that mindfulness is like the oil in an engine: We can drive the car for a while when it's low, but often when we've been driving it hard and then need it the most, the engine is destined to fuse and completely break down. Being mindful of the level of the oil and seeing to the engine's regular needs produce the greatest health for that which drives our organizations. This requires a level of awareness that we refer to as "being here now."

The Root of Relationship

At the heart of awareness and of all relationships, for that matter, is our ability to be here now—not to be distracted from where we are and the work of the moment. But how does one introduce this idea into an organization that has never experienced it before? It is a job that must begin with the leadership of an organization. Unfortunately, when we lock ourselves deeper and deeper into a mind-filled state, we often don't know that there are other alternatives to the "normal" we've created. We become blind to the existence of what health is and can be.

What we see is that the level at which an organization can be here now determines the effectiveness of everything it does. It's the dimension that makes systems, policies, and procedures work more effectively. It also allows people to respond appropriately to the challenges and issues they encounter, rather than just react. And most importantly, it provides the space to discover the direction necessary to move into the future as a force in industry and the community. How does it do so?

When we are present now, mindful of the world in which we are living, we are capable of accessing greater wisdom. The good news is, this mindful state that delivers so much is not something we have to learn how to do. It is what we refer to as our "default setting," and all it requires is our willingness to access it. In the mindful state, we exhibit the behaviors of be here now. We also find all the same things that we strive for with a filled mind, but they look very different. In a mind-filled state, compassion, for instance, looks either like tolerance or patience and wisdom looks something akin to intellect or cleverness. In a mindful state, compassion and understanding might revolve around being here now for others and ourselves, and wisdom is a receptivity to what is unknown. The mind-filled state is less forgiving and more superficial. One may ask, "But why do I need compassion and wisdom in business?" The ability to access our innate wisdom and compassion is of tremendous value to any organization because it is the source of every relational activity, and business, at its core, is relating and interacting.

So are we attempting to create a perfect organization without problems? The reality is a Mindful Corporation often encounters the same problems facing less-healthy organizations, but those problems are just not viewed in the same way nor do they have the same effect or implications within a company. All companies face competitive forces, changes in technology, shifts in the economy and industry, employee issues, production glitches, and occasional sabotage. The answer is in keeping one's bearings and dealing with these issues with wisdom and sensitivity. Being mindful doesn't remove the problems that we face. It just allows us to face those problems more consciously as an integral part of life. As people access their wisdom more, they accept both the positive and the negative with a tremendous amount of flexibility, receptivity, and understanding.

The Tennessee Valley Authority's Bill Thompson believes the underlying strength here is one of resiliency: "If people are more personally resilient in a rapidly changing environment, that organization is going to handle change with a lot more gracefulness and ease. All of us have had the experience in which we resisted a change, but in the end it worked out for the better. Our own internal mental battles degraded our performance in life, or enjoyment of life, and for nothing."

Often, people gain this understanding very late in life, and some only while on their deathbed. It is here they realize that they are going to miss everything that life offers, both the good news and the bad. They recognize at that moment that what they thought was the bad part was all part of the wonderful experience of life and it was all worth living.

So how does this translate into the real world? Let us look at the case of Dick Abdoo, the CEO of Wisconsin Electric, who had to make some rather difficult decisions regarding a sensitive situation. A child was playing where he should not have and he found his way into a neighborhood electrical transformer. The lock had broken off and he squiggled in and was electrocuted. It wasn't that this transformer was simply open and flapping in the breeze for all who walked by to see. The boy had to climb over two fences to get in there, but it was still a terrible situation. But rather than closing ranks and becoming insecure and protected, the CEO remained open, tapped into his wisdom, and assumed complete accountability for what happened. This was contrary to all the suggestions that he received from his senior team, his bank of attorneys, and the board of directors. They were advising him to lay low and let the attorneys fight it out in court. But he wouldn't have it. That was "normal" business and he wouldn't do it. He went on the airwaves and took accountability for the situation. He said that he had met with the parents of the child and together they had settled the issue, and Wisconsin Electric would not shirk its responsibility. In coming from his integrity, the CEO dealt mindfully and wisely with the situation, without regard to outcome. In doing so, the community and the company rallied behind him, and the traumatic impact on both the family and the organization was greatly minimized.

Upon reflection, had he not acted from his wisdom and integrity at that moment, the cost to all concerned would have been far greater both emotionally and financially. His healthy response allowed the community to begin to heal as well as to see what can happen when we are mindful of our relationship to the world in which we operate. The people in his organization were also impacted, being reminded of their own state of health, and as a result, began acting more mindfully. They treated each other with greater respect and the quality of service they provided to the community improved.

In creating the Mindful Corporation, all we are doing is developing an organization that is more aware of and accountable to the world in which it operates. And by that awareness, something very simple takes place. The organization becomes healthier, and in the eyes of all of those who view it, more successful. People are always attracted to health because it is something that lives within them as a default setting, and they recognize it as the core goodness we all contain that is impervious to our experience. It resonates in them as being innate, whether or not they are currently living it. Next we will discuss how our health comes into being and the distractions that keep us from it; i.e., the role of thinking and how it drives the vital operations of our lives.

Chapter Three

The Role of Thought

"Thought is not reality; yet it is through Thought that our realities are created. It is what we as humans put into our thoughts that dictates what we think of life."

—

Sidney Banks

No matter *what* we think, there is no escaping the fact *that* we think. Everything we do is preceded by a thought; our ability to form images in our minds. But there is a distinction to be made between the content of thought and the process of thought—this is the difference between *what* we think and *that* we think. It is when we understand the idea *that* we think, we find greater health and fulfillment.

To better understand this, let's take the image of a coffee cup. In this regard, we are talking about the cup, not what the cup holds. The nature of the liquid in the cup is its content; the cup itself is the process of thought. For example, perhaps we find ourselves either feeling bad or good toward a person. If we were to focus on the content of thought, the avenue we would take would be to ask ourselves why we feel bad. What are the thoughts we're holding that made us feel this particular way toward this person? That is all content. Thought content is captured in what we think about our biases, memories, beliefs, convictions, opinions, and impressions. It is how we see a situation or what we make of it. It is our understanding of things, people, and events. Just as this description helps make sense of this idea, so, too, content helps us make sense of the world. It seems to provide us with a sense of security to know what is going on around us or that we can predict the future and its outcomes. It is easy to imagine why we would try to work with the content. There is an illusion of progress toward understanding in this approach. Often, people achieve some degree of perspective on the content of their thinking, some distance to better see what they are looking at. But as that description suggests, it's not the content that they are coming to grips with; it's the perspective, which is part of the process of thought. In this regard, perspective is *how* we think and content is *what* we think.

In a business setting, leading someone toward perspective and away from content becomes extremely important for improving relationships. This is especially true between team members. The reason is simple: When people have perspective, when they can step back from entanglements and recognize their thinking and that of others, they don't get caught in each other's content or memories. When this is avoided, people can work well together, and better, more productive ideas emerge as do more productive relationships.

Let us provide an example of what takes place when we come from both of these places, each approach beginning with content. Suppose we're speaking with Ralph who tells us, "I don't get along with Sam."

From a content approach we might reply, "Why is that?"

"Well, he's sneaky."

"When was the first time you felt that way?" Again, we're addressing the content of the situation, not Ralph's process. So we try to figure out a way to discount the content by asking, "Is his sneakiness a fact or is it your imagination?"

The reply might be, "It's fact." Then Ralph would tell his story about how he trusted Sam to do one thing, but he actually did the exact opposite. When he spoke to Sam about it, Sam said he knew what he was doing, but he went ahead and did it anyway.

So, when discounting the content doesn't work, we might try to teach Ralph coping mechanisms—how to cope with his "dysfunctional" thought. Then, if that doesn't work, we might teach him how to reframe his thinking so that he is actually trying to trick his thought with another thought. If that doesn't work, we teach him strategizing techniques to minimize the possible negative impact of the content; his mistrust of Sam. In actuality, all we are doing is adding effort and business to Ralph's life, as well as validating his original thought of Sam's sneakiness.

If we focus on the process of thought, the differences may appear subtle, but the outcome can be profound. In the same situation, Ralph says to us, "I just can't trust Sam."

We ask, "Why is that?" We'd hear the same story. But instead of getting stuck in the content, we might tell him something like, "We all have good days and bad days. We're at the top of our game sometimes, and other times we are at the bottom. Some days we feel full of life, and other days we feel very insecure." Then we might ask, "Do you interact with Sam frequently?"

"Yes, I have to; we are kind of locked at the hip on this project," would come the reply.

"Well, has he screwed you every time you've done something together?"

"Not every time, but I'm keeping my eye on him. I'm really being defensive because the moment I take my eye off him, he'll probably screw me again."

"That's always a possibility, but have you ever dropped the ball or let someone down or did something that you had to apologize for?"

"Yeah."

"Do you do it all the time?"

"No."

"Why not? Is it because someone is keeping his eye on you?"

"No. When I did do it, I was very frightened or insecure. But for the most part, I can keep my bearings."

"Well, let's just entertain this possibility: Do you think that the same thing might apply in varying degrees with Sam?"

At the very least, he might begrudgingly admit, "Well, maybe."

That's enough of a seam to start teaching Ralph about thought. Not what he thinks, but *that* he thinks. All the different aspects of his feelings toward Sam are affected by his thinking. By explaining this, all we are doing is giving him perspective.

Our perception of reality determines our reaction to it. Our perception of reality is determined by our thoughts of the events and situations in our lives. Perspective comes from the distance we get via recognizing the role thought plays in our interpretation of those events. Therefore, our effectiveness in life and our workplace is determined by our relationship with thought—not its content. In other words, *that* we think is more valuable to us and our relationships than *what* we think.

Recognizing Levels of Understanding

Perspective also provides us with the opportunity to recognize our current level of understanding. In our work, we often represent this idea on a vertical chart.

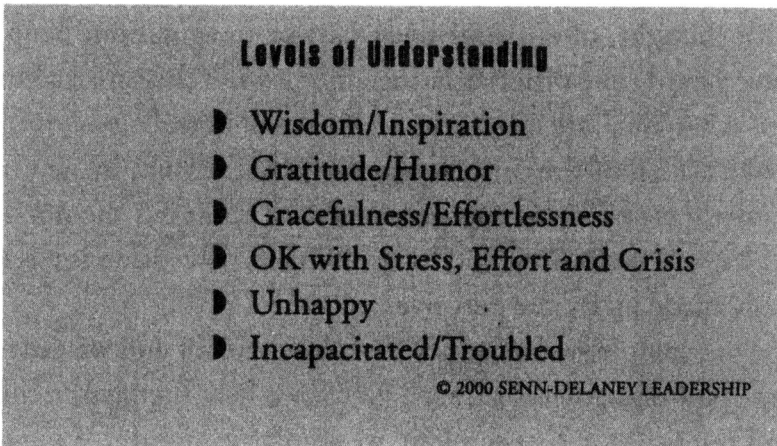

Levels of Understanding

▶ Wisdom/Inspiration
▶ Gratitude/Humor
▶ Gracefulness/Effortlessness
▶ OK with Stress, Effort and Crisis
▶ Unhappy
▶ Incapacitated/Troubled

© 2000 SENN-DELANEY LEADERSHIP

While we list only six different levels here, it is important to acknowledge that there are really infinite levels in this progression. The basic idea here is that life is not a static plane of understanding as it may appear, but is available to be experienced at different levels. Each successive level up this continuum is more profound, gentler, and more impactive. Imagine this figure filled with levels above and below each of the levels noted. What we will provide, however, is a way to experience the thinking behind each of these six levels.

The lowest level of understanding we've experienced in business—where the business is still "in operation" although flirting with bankruptcy—is *troubled, incapacitated, highly fearful,* or *tremendously angry.* The feelings and manifestations associated with this troubled level of understanding are a function of the thinking of the people in the organization. This is the mind-filled organization at its most mind-filled state. As might be expected, the mind-filled organization is filled with mind-filled individuals. When the mind is so filled with thought, often from one's past or imagination, people have a hard time differentiating among what they are making up, what they are perceiving, and what is real. Everything looks real all of the time. It should be noted, that by its very nature, perception is composed of such things as memories, biases, and prejudices, and so, as thought, perception is essentially made up by the perceiver.

For example, we're walking by a house plant and we hear it say, "Kill that guy over there." What we hear the plant tell us and our walking by the plant are similar in nature. We can't differentiate between reality and imagination. Sometimes, imagination causes the most harm. Suppose on our way home we start imagining, "The plant must know more than I do." This happens in a blink of an eye. It is not something that just comes over us. Then, the moment we notice the foolishness of our thoughts, as opposed to taking them seriously, we step into a higher plane of health. We might say,

"Wait a minute here. Plants can't talk." The moment we experience that degree of perspective, we are in a higher level of understanding. The mind-filled person sees no difference between what they perceive as reality and what they make of it. They don't recognize the role their thoughts play in their perception of reality.

Moving Up the Continuum

The next level is the unhappy or defensive level. There is more perspective here than in the troubled level, but because of the amount of insecurity present, people stuck in this level are usually playing "not to lose" rather than "to win." They are very defensive, which makes complete sense to them because they are only seeing what is wrong rather than what is right.

There is a world of difference between seeing what is wrong and what could be better. In the first level, the way people get away from the pain caused by their thinking is through escapism—either through alcoholism or drugs, through emotional or physical abuse, or by vilifying the people or situations in which they become involved. The second level of understanding is a bit more socially correct, but the way people release energy from their thinking, the way they let steam off at this level, is by complaining a lot. They always see the dark side of things. "Don't trust" is often their mantra. When we listen to people who are always complaining or worrying, we know they are at this level of defensiveness or insecurity.

Now, the bottom two levels we're discussing here certainly do exist, but 90 percent of the organizations we see fall into the next level in which life is OK, but there are certain prices we have to pay for that "OKness." This translates into effort, living in a world of stress, dealing with occasional crises, or in some cases, going from crisis to crisis. We see a great deal of people who, if they don't have crisis, create crisis. They always do it for very good reasons, perhaps to prove that they are good people, or that they have value within the organization or community.

For example, we know one person who is constantly bringing either drug addicts or alcoholics into his home. We'll call him Bob. He is like a social magnet for these folks. Bob goes from person to person; when one upsets him he gets rid of them. He says things like, "I couldn't trust him; he kept stealing things." It's not much of a surprise. Bob brings a drug addict into his home who steals things and sells them to buy more drugs. Bob feels, "He should have had more respect for me and my home." When asked who's taking the drug addict's bedroom, Bob answers, "I found a guy who was expelled from school and was kicked out of his parents' house."

The fact is, Bob takes these people in for "good reasons," to be of service, but his life then is hectic, busy, and always has a tale to tell. There is a world of difference between Bob and the person who is doing deeds like this out of a true sense of service. The person who is acting out of true service, from an inside-out perspective, does so without concern for outside return or expectation. This person has understanding and patience and rarely wears them like a "red badge of courage" because he or she is capable of gaining a healthy perspective on their situation.

In the workplace, the effort extended in the "OK, but" level could be anything from constantly attending self-help seminars to going on vacations. This is also where coping mechanisms come into play. At this level of OK, we find seminars dealing with topics like coping with stress, anger management, adjusting your world, and behavior modification. Relationship improvement programs are prevalent, and people are searching everywhere for ways of making things easier. About 75 percent of what we understand at this level is that life can be OK, but it takes effort, and there is a good chance that things must be done in a certain way.

Many people, at one point in time, come to the heartfelt realization that life is an inside-out phenomenon, not outside-in. The first three levels of understanding that we described—troubled, unhappy, and OK—are all about how to cope with seeing life as outside-in, how we deal with life as it shows up. That is, how we feel inside is determined by what is going on outside of us through situations and events. If someone frowns at us, we should feel bad. If we don't hit our targets or our goals, we should feel insecure or our self-esteem should be diminished.

Of course, the opposite side of the coin is also outside-in, as when our self-esteem is linked to hitting our goals. We hit them, and our self-esteem goes up. Unfortunately, this rise in self-esteem is short-lived and when accompanied by some strutting and patting oneself on the back, can often look a lot like arrogance. There is usually little humility associated with this perspective, and, as such, the seeds of its demise are inherent in how long this outer-driven self-esteem can be fed.

Being stuck in the content of thought or what we are thinking limits our possibilities and makes everything more difficult. When we begin to notice the process of thought, we immediately step into a higher level of understanding above an imaginary line between good health and poor health. The first level of good health is the world of gracefulness. It is a world in which things seem to happen naturally with ease and effortlessness. We feel as if we're in the groove, what athletes refer to as "the zone." Life seems to move easily, and we begin noticing the process of thought rather than its content. We might find that while working on a project, time seems to pass unnoticed with the right information seemingly at our fingertips. Fatigue is not an issue. Our perspective and patience increase greatly. When something happens that would have at one time set us off, we recognize that it was our thinking that caused us to go off, and we react without upset. We are easily contented. As a matter of fact, we are often as content with the small and simple as we are with the great because our contentment is not being driven from outside ourselves, but rather from our own state of mind. We discover that our working relationships happen easily. They are not something to worry about or force into being different than what they are. As a result, decisions are made more easily because we are capable of getting beyond the places at which we might habitually have gotten stuck if we didn't recognize our thought. In fact, not only are decisions easier, but the quality of decisions are much better since we have more facile access to our innate wisdom. When people are moving through their day at a level of gracefulness, they find their zone more easily, enjoy themselves more, and appreciate where they are in life.

As our understanding rises to the next level, we frequently find ourselves full of gratitude and humor. When we operate out of this level, effortlessness and gracefulness are a matter of course. We realize that gratefulness is nothing more than a state of mind out of which we can operate, and we find we are grateful for a lot more than just the effortlessness and gracefulness of life. We see life with a capital "L," appreciating all it has to offer, not just the good. Everything is in perspective. We are not driven by it, but see where, in fact, we can be of service and how we can contribute. When operating at this level, we appear to others to be in the right place at the right time.

At the top of our continuum is the highest level we have ever seen: wisdom and inspiration. There are undoubtedly higher levels, but this is the highest we know of. People who live at a level of wisdom and inspiration appear to display foresight; an uncanny ability to see around corners. So far, those who operate at this level are very rare. This is a level often associated with enlightenment or living the innate.

From a business perspective, this becomes interesting when we realize that where we are on the level of understanding continuum impacts how we see the world. For example, when a company publishes its values, such as, "We will operate with respect and trust toward one another," the way this will be perceived varies on one's level of understanding. At the lowest level, we might hear something like, "How dare they try to jam their stuff into my life. What gives them the right to do it?" Then, moving up the continuum a bit more, we might hear, "I will when they start doing it." A little higher up…"What's in it for me?" A little higher up… "It's just the flavor of the month. I'm going to hang around for the kick-off. I'm bound to get a bonus out of it." A little higher up would be, "If they want me to act this way, they have to pay me more."

Those individuals who recognize that their thinking determines their perception of reality also bring a great deal of perspective to what appears to happen to them. We would hear things like, "Isn't that interesting that senior management is concerned about quality of life. I thought they were only interested in bottom-line results." A little higher up, "These are all wonderful ideas. They are certainly worthy of my effort." A little higher up would be, "You know what, I'd like to make this a better place for not only myself but for my friends and co-workers." A little higher up would be "You know if I could make this work at XYZ company, I wonder if we could do something similar within the community in which I live?"

It doesn't matter what is said or the accuracy of the words chosen. The level of understanding of the individuals who perceive the words determines how a communication is heard. As mentioned above, it also determines how any event is perceived, or even more to the point, that events are often neutral, but we still have the ability to view an event in a variety of ways. In addition, the level of understanding of those communicating the words can also have a positive effect. Volunteers of America's Bob Pratt suggests that "As you start being different, people start getting curious about you being different, 'Why are you happy?' 'Why are you calmer?' It's almost viral. Once people are experiencing you differently, in a very positive sense from their perspective, they simply want to know more about being different themselves. It's not something you have to talk to them about. It resonates."

It's All Viewpoint

What Pratt is alluding to is that how a person views life determines how they go through life—how productive they are, their energy level, their focus, and whether they contribute in a positive or negative fashion. As Ron Adams explains it, "There are times when I can move effortlessly with a lot of pace and there are other days when I am just fighting it. The only difference is me."

Organizations, in an effort to get their people more productive or to improve their attitude, have innocently enforced methods of motivation to get people to produce. Not too surprisingly, the results are different at each level of understanding. In organizations operating at the lowest level where people are troubled and incapacitated, motivation is couched with threats and fear. We hear managers say things like, "If you can't get it done, I'm sure I can find someone who will." "There are more people to do your job than just you."

At the level of unhappy, motivation is often approached from a point of view of obligation or guilt. We run into this level of unhappy quite frequently when there has been a recent downsizing. The heaviness of responsibility and guilt are often used to motivate the remaining employees. There are lots of "victim" stories at this level. The thinking is often, "If you are a good person, you'll do it." And, "If you don't do it, you are a 'bad' person."

At the level of OK, we find rewards and recognition. In and of itself, recognition is not debilitating. But when viewed from this level of understanding, recognition becomes an ego-based desire and lure that can be used as a bargaining chip to influence one's self-esteem, sense of worth, and impressions of justice. All of this is still appealing to the individual who sees things from the outside in. It appears to work because the mindset is an outside-in mindset. At the level of effortlessness and gracefulness, however, motivation becomes an inside-out feeling of common sense—"Well, of course, I do this not because I expect something, but because I am motivated from within to do what I know is right." Often at this level, discussions and dialogues are much easier because what is listened for is the grain of truth in the conversation, not necessarily who said what to whom. Breakthroughs occur at this level of perception.

At the level of gratitude and humor, motivation appears as a true sense of service, not only with clients, but also with co-workers and community. This is a place of synergy where often it doesn't take as much discussion to move forward as it does at the previous, lower level. As we go higher above the line, we find ourselves more and more in the moment and much less being tied to yesterday. What we have been told is that at the highest level, there is a sense of shared vision—not how the vision manifests itself, but the shared vision of the feeling that lies behind the vision. If this sounds confusing, that's because this is a state, much like the Zen state, that defies description. It is an intimate experience of what precedes thought.

Let's think about just the movement up this vertical dimension of understanding. At the lower levels, we are either the beneficiary or the victim of circumstance. It is very much an outside-in world. At the middle levels, we are aware of thought, but are coming from a place where we are trying to control the content. We experience different degrees of self-consciousness. This level is where we find a proliferation of rules to remind us how to behave. Techniques abound to help us cope or maximize the situation. However, lurking in the shadows is the specter of judgment, for oneself as well as toward others.

In the higher levels or states, the healing, wisdom, and answers occur in a very natural way. Instead of focusing on thought or its content, we open ourselves to that which precedes thought. The moment we experience this birthplace of thought, life happens. This is very difficult to conceptualize because we are not describing a physical location out of which thought arises, rather, what Eastern thought has often referred to as "formlessness." Prayer is actually a good example. At the lower level, we pray for God to give us things. In the middle level, we pray for God to guide us. At the upper levels, we are more at one with life and our prayers are often those of gratitude and appreciation, not a physical entreaty.

A basic premise behind the Mindful Corporation is that at any given moment our perceptions can change. We are not saying make the "best" of how we see reality, but that reality itself completely changes. We have been referring to this phenomenon as a shift in understanding.

The conduit between perception and reality is thought. As such, the quality of our thought has a direct influence on the quality of our experience. Commensurately, our response, decision, and actions are a result of this quality. If we want greater effectiveness, fulfillment, and service, we must raise the quality of our thoughts.

Raising the quality of our thoughts is not something we do; it's something we allow. Imagine the many ways our thinking manifests itself: memory recall, analysis, compassion, humor, wisdom, common sense, inspiration, foresight, and hindsight. Our ability to access all of those things really determines the quality of the decisions that we make. If we could access our full range of capacities more of the time, then we would make more effective decisions. If we were to do this, the odds would also be in our favor for operating a more successful company.

The Modes of Thought

In its simplest form, we have two modes of thinking that allow us to actualize these capacities. We call them *forced mode* and *flow mode*. Forced mode gives us the illusion of control. We have the sense that we can force high-quality thinking within ourselves. In doing so, however, we limit ourselves to a marginal amount of memory recall, impose the effort of the analysis process, and suffer reduced creativity. The feelings attached to this forced-mode way of thinking also differ from flow mode. Actions are more effortful, rather than allowing the thought to occur. We are more arrogant than humble, impatient rather than quiet, and judgmental rather than evaluative. In this mode of thinking, we tend to limit ourselves to what has happened or been previously thought in the entire spectrum of past, present, and future.

An example of the difference in quality between the two modes would be the difference between forcing a golf drive and allowing it to happen while in the "zone." The first is memory driven. We swing with all our might, trying to remember all the things we've been taught. Invariably, the quality of the swing can be limited and unreliable, especially as we watch the ball dribble off the tee. When we're in flow mode, we simply step up and power the ball down the fairway.

In the business environment, forced mode is when we

become more self-conscious about our actions and attempt to exert greater self-control. There is a tinge of insecurity, pressure, tension and possibly anger to forced mode. In both flow and forced mode, we may think analytically as we process thought, but the feeling and quality between "flow" and "forced" differs. Anything in life can be done in forced mode; it is just more effortful and usually accomplished with less joy.

From the perspective of organizations, we have found that forced thinking fills the mind quickly. Flow mode is a more spacious and mindful approach. The reality is that few, if any, people operate totally in flow mode. We constantly find ourselves moving back and forth between the two.

In addition to flow mode and forced mode, we also want to differentiate between the mode of thought and the function of thought. In forced mode, we are often conscious of how we are thinking. In flow mode, that self-conscious quality falls away. We're not aware of how we are thinking. The moment we think about being in flow mode, we are no longer in it. We can think about forced mode and still be in it. We are more aware of what we are thinking. Flow mode thinking just happens. We notice it after the fact and can't prepare for it before the fact. We can prepare for forced mode, though we can't prepare for flow mode. We can anticipate forced mode, but there's no anticipating when we will enter flow mode. All we can do is be prepared to do so. And unfortunately, as mentioned previously, once we're there and we become conscious of being there, we're no longer in it.

We know we are locked in forced mode when there is too much to consider for the conscious mind to deal with—or stated differently, when we are mind-filled. Intuitively, what do we do when the mind becomes filled and conscious of its thinking? We either quiet it all down or simply move on to something else.

Now, moving on to something else may sound like a first-class avoidance of the work ethic. We have been taught to focus until we solve the problem. But a much healthier approach, and one that actually is more efficient and realizes faster results, is that if we can't come up with an answer to our problem in a few minutes, then we should move on to something else. As long as the flow of thoughts feels fresh or the conversation is moving forward, keep at it. This is an example of how wonderfully designed we are as human beings. If we were moving ahead nicely, we simply stay in that flow state. But, if we're struggling and forcing through our thoughts and nothing is coming, we're defeating our purpose if we continue. What happens? The moment we move on to something else, we invariably get an insight into our original problem. Most people have a difficult time accepting this. They feel they have to forge ahead. But when we ask them, "When did you come up with the idea?" We find the response is usually, "When I let go and took a deep breath." The reality is they probably could have taken that step toward release hours earlier.

By forcing the issue, our minds become mind-filled, thick with our own thoughts, and we tend to get lost in the minutia.

So if flow mode is so wonderful, what keeps us from always being in it? Or, do we even want to always be in flow? To repeat ourselves, it would be truly amazing for someone to be in a state of constant flow mode. Self-consciousness, self desire, goal setting, ego, insecurity, arrogance, the need for control, and the illusion of predetermination are all mind-filled thoughts that keep us in a forced rather than flow mode. The majority of us can't get away from the way we have fashioned life. Many think they could do life quite nicely and never be in flow mode. It's all part of what we have grown accustomed to. It may not feel good, but it is familiar.

How do our organizations operate differently when we interact in and out of this flow state? This is the great potential of the Mindful Corporation. When people in flow mode interact, the wisdom that emerges out of that interaction is greater, more directed, and creative. It can't be otherwise. Why? Because people in flow know that a thought blockage is not the time to press harder, but the time to release. Once the blockage moves on, the answer emerges without all the wasted effort tied to trying to surmount the temporary log-jam of our thoughts. That makes for a much more productive use of everyone's time.

As with concepts like enlightenment and self-realization, we can only really discuss flow mode to a given point, because as its name implies, it doesn't lend itself to the notion of form. This is difficult for some to understand because we were brought up in a world of making sense only out of those things that have form. Flow mode does not fit into that mold. We can talk about its manifestations, but the moment we put form on it is the moment we lose it. Such is the nature of the Mindful Corporation; we are unable to put limits on it. Every time we try to do so, we limit what is possible and we move into a reactive forced mode of thinking. As Plato said over 2500 years ago, "We are in a process of everlasting becoming."

Once we have become, once we are, the flow stops.

Within the context of this book, we can offer some of the manifestations an organization capable of operating in flow mode can expect, the profound impact of these manifestations on our interactions and relationships, and the product of those encounters. The English mathematician and philosopher Alfred North Whitehead made the point that "Orthodox experiments reveal orthodox novelty." Flow mode leaves the constriction of orthodox thinking behind and allows us to enter the new. And because we have greater perspective in flow mode, we are able to keep our bearings when we are confronted by something unexpected. When we find ourselves in those unanticipated areas, perspective allows us patience and clarity. We may also discover that the simplest things touch and move us.

Recognizing Our Thinking

The creation of the Mindful Corporation process begins with our ability to recognize our thinking. For some, we may not realize the level of our thoughts until well after we have acted. Others may see their thinking right after they do something. At that place, thought recognition is not about content, it is the simple observance that we think and that there is a source of thought that precedes the thought itself. But before we can experience the source of thought, we have to first recognize that we are thinking. Then we have to let go of that recognition to move on to the experience of the source.

Now this may sound arcane and convoluted, but it's really quite logical. The idea of thought recognition is fairly simple. If we stop for a moment and sit quietly, our minds take off and thoughts almost immediately rise up, even if that thought is "Why am I sitting here listening to my thoughts?" We can't just turn off the fact that we think.

Once we realize that we think, we've already taken the next step to get to the source of thought. So what does that mean? First of all, many people don't even realize they think, much less recognize the role their thinking plays in their construct of life and their circumstances. They know they are thinking creatures, but they don't know they think. They don't know their own thought place. They think it is all just a lot of mumbo-jumbo. It's inconsequential; "Okay, so I think. Tell me what I should do."

Getting to the Bus Stop

By its very definition, we can't consciously make flow mode happen, or force access to it. We can notice when we are not there. Metaphorically, all we can do is get ourselves to the bus stop, but we can't guarantee the bus will be there, or if and when it is scheduled to arrive. We do know that we can't get on the bus without being at the bus stop. And once we notice we are on the bus, it slows down and we get off. Mental still-ness seems to provide our only clue to the bus approaching.

Now there are those who will readily say, "How is this going to be helpful in my business if I never know when I am going to get on and I never know when I am going to be getting off?"

The reason it is helpful in business is to prevent us from spending more time or making important decisions when we are off the bus. What we are not suggesting is to walk around noticing when we are not in flow mode. The only reason we are presenting this is that at our present level of understanding, we know that the quality of the decisions and our interactions are suspect when our thoughts come from insecurity or forced mode. The moment we have the perspective to notice that, we are stepping into flow mode. It is that we notice it and we step in that direction. When we find ourselves deep in the middle of thinking about where we are, we are deep in the middle of forced mode.

Getting Beyond Making It Happen

Since many of us can't get beyond our need to control or surrender to the idea that we can't make something happen, this journey we are describing may seem very foreign.

All we hear at work is "Make it happen." All we think is, "I make it happen and that is why I am successful." We are not suggesting that we are unimportant in the game of life. We still do life, and there are arenas in life where we can make things happen and over which we can have influence—how we raise our kids, how we do our job, how we interact within our community. But when it comes to accessing the full range of the capacities of our thinking, we simply cannot make flow happen. We can't make our people more positive or more open to change. While we can provide the right circumstances, we cannot force the last step. That is purely their choice.

What we gain within our organization by having this ability to get on the bus of flow mode is that we make better decisions. Because of our awareness of flow, we quickly notice when we are mentally hectic and off base. This, in itself, is significant because, as stated earlier, when we are not here now, we don't make the best decisions for the organization.

The impact of better and more innovative decisions arising out of our wisdom, rather than relying on decisions based solely on memory, is what fuels healthy growth.

Business has traditionally made an errant assumption: that we can force performance. Better performance doesn't happen because we will it so. If that were the case, we wouldn't spend billions searching for answers to improving performance. It occurs because of our innate capabilities to be here now and operate in flow. When a leader is present with an employee, listening and engaging from a flow perspective, the employee feels heard and the opportunity for change takes place. Gunn Partner's CEO Bob Gunn thinks the key to this openness is listening. "What listening gives us," he says, "is insight. Listening in a group process multiplies the insight of any one individual. So, when people are listening really deeply, we can feel the power in that because of the depth of understanding that happens out of that deep listening. The listening actually gives us clarity about what to do."

This is not some illusive, fickle process. We do not need to make an effort to be in flow, we only have to be ready to get on the bus. Intuitively, we know this is true. That is, we perform better when we are in a healthy state of mind. Our instinct might then tell us, if this is true, "Let's make sure we're always in a healthy flow." But, once we start forcing others or ourselves into that state, we diminish our health and are quickly led astray or we expend energy in a worthwhile endeavor that ultimately is a fruitless cause.

Now, the fact that we can't force our flow may be difficult to buy if we are at the level of understanding that says such things as "I do the influencing. No pain, no gain. Anything worth doing is worth doing with effort." That is how many of us were brought up, and it hasn't changed a great deal over the years. The problem we find with that way of thinking is that it takes a great deal of effort to live life in that fashion.

This does not mean we can't determine what we want to do or what direction we want to head. Once we have done that, we put ourselves at the bus stop and are ready to get on. George Pransky once said there was a reason why Albert Einstein didn't come up with great football plays: That wasn't his direction. Once we determine direction, the whole idea is to put ourselves in a place ready to access our high-quality thoughts to assist us in moving in that direction.

Putting It to Work

This is not a laissez faire, *ca sera, sera* life approach. It is very purposeful. We are opening ourselves to more possibilities that may be surprising, but they are ultimately healthier for the organization than those made otherwise. One example of this by an executive we know at a major banking institution was especially surprising to his higher-ups. He had gone through this process and realized his ultimate responsibility to the organization was to provide the greatest value to their shareholders. This thought was about much more than making sense. It came from his very personal vision—his *raison d'etre*—his reason for being of service to all he served. This is an example of what we call an act of "corporate citizenship." When he took a look at his organization, he realized that there was a much better way of doing what he did. There was a tremendous amount of redundancy and millions of dollars being spent, unnecessarily.

He had an organization of 5,000 people involved primarily in information technology. His problem was one of responsiveness; being able to change the nature of information technology within the organization and getting it to the field appropriately. When an organization is trying to be the leader in its field, the importance of this is obvious. He went to his boss and said, "The way we are structured right now is like a bank. What we need is to be structured like the companies in Silicon Valley. Here is what I recommend. I maintain a small group of 500 people that keep in touch with the latest technological advancements. That is our mission. But, for the remaining 4,500 people, we have them report to the people they support. "

His boss couldn't believe it, but went to the corporation and said, "This is not my idea. In fact, I tried to talk him out of it, because politically it makes no sense. He is downsizing his organization to one-tenth of what it was. But, for the good of the organization, here is what he recommended." As with his boss, the corporation did not believe that anybody in their right mind would put the service of the corporation first, rather than trying to increase his or her own power. Nonetheless, they did it, and the change worked brilliantly. The executive did what was healthiest for the organization and everyone ultimately benefited. This is the kind of thought that can only arise in flow mode. Flow ideas fly in the face of what we have been taught and are often counterintuitive. The vast majority of the people cannot believe that anybody would do that "in their right mind."

Once this leader let go of all his constrictive thoughts of success, of how he was supposed to play the corporate game, this new thought started to take on more meaning for him. As he described it, "I thought I would be really fearful about only having 500 people. I was a senior corporate executive. I thought I would be much more insecure not having this massive organization wrapped around me. But I'm not."

When we become aware of the thoughts and feelings that keep us out of flow mode, answers can arise that are often unexpected and that better benefit the organization in total. Why? Because these ideas can only arise from a higher level of understanding. If the company is worthwhile, imagine what would happen if every employee, from the CEO on down, were open to the thoughts and actions of what was best for the company and its constituents.

The most obvious impediments we encounter from keeping this image are being frightened or feeling insecure, questioning ourselves, seeing bogeymen in other people, and seeing traps and layers everywhere. If that is the nature of our world, then we have to expect that our decisions are going to be somewhat flawed because of that perspective. If we notice that life is taking on much more of a hum-drum familiarity to it—"This year I have more to do and I have higher targets, but primarily, with that exception, this year is no different than last"—we have just experienced another indication that our decision will only produce more of the same.

The Mindful Corporation is not one in which gurus are leading each and every department. But once this philosophy is integrated throughout an organization, those who resist operating from a healthy perspective stand out more and more. If they stay energized, many of them will become healthier because of the influence of those around them.

When healthiness is too scary for an individual because of their level of understanding, they leave. Usually, for these people everything is threatening.

We often see this in personal relationships. When a person goes from failed relationship to failed relationship, it is usually because they are repeating an unhealthy pattern. They blame the content of the relationship for its failure, not their process of relating. Sooner or later they will have to face this, because it keeps coming back at them until they do. Or, they simply resign themselves to the fact that they will never have a successful relationship. Instead of defending or ignoring how life presents itself, the first step in resolving issues like these is for a person to truly "accept their lot in life." As author Pema Chodron suggests, "Start where you are." Once a person can come to peace with where they are, and treat themselves gently in so doing, then, and only then, can they move forward gracefully.

The whole concept of the Mindful Corporation is built on the evolution of the mindful individual, which in turn, is given power and a sense of urgency by the mindful leader. Leaders can create a culture that fosters the ability to understand and recognize the role of thought throughout an organization by their actions and thereby, hopefully, create more mindful and reflective people. In turn, this builds a greater perspective and wisdom for the organization in relation to what they do and decide, and most powerfully, a mindful understanding creates and maintains a synergy with others, both within and without the company.

We see this most prominently reflected in meetings. When we recognize our thinking and the source of those thoughts, listening immediately improves greatly. We also gain all the benefits from listening, including the elimination of the machinations when listening doesn't occur. There is also less arguing and much more dialogue. Decisions are also reached more quickly. While we discuss this in greater detail in Chapter 7, when people are mindful, they leave meetings in greater alignment so there are less pocket vetoes, thus dispelling hidden agendas. These gatherings become more effective and people look forward to them rather than being a source of dread and a waste of valuable time.

The Bottom Line is a Thought, Too

What we have found is that a mindful approach directly improves the bottom line. Because we are able to make better quality decisions, our organizations operate more cohesively, with alignment and common purpose. We will discuss the power of aligned interactions in Chapter 8, but each of these issues plays out on the bottom line. If we were to speak with just about any CEO and start peeling back the onion regarding what bottom-line issues his or her company has, no matter if it's "our margins are shrinking, our sales are decreasing, we're not keeping pace with the competition," it all eventually gets back to the role of thought within the organization. Santa Fe Institute economist Brian Arthur has said that all business failures are cognitive, that is, they are a failure of our thinking. James Champy has also said, "People like to think that businesses are built of numbers (as in the 'bottom line'), or forces (as in 'market forces'), or things ('the product'), or even flesh and blood ('our people'). But this is wrong…Businesses are made of ideas—ideas expressed as words."

This is why we believe so strongly that an organization that encourages its people to be more mindful and conscious of the health out of which it operates can't fail. Why do we feel so confident in making that statement? If we think about it for a moment, it makes sense. When we reduce politicking—hold on to fewer grudges with less positioning and posturing—practice increased listening, support, and alignment; work with each other with greater mutual respect and understanding (which in turn creates greater self-esteem and fulfillment); take quicker, more accurate actions; and make better and faster decisions, the results can only be positive.

Chapter Four

Slowing It Down To Run Faster

"Being caught up in a strong consuming mood is a roadblock to smooth interaction. If we enter into a conversation while preoccupied by a strong mood, the other person is likely to experience us as being unavailable, or what the sociologist Irving Goffman has called 'away'—just going through the motions of the conversation while obviously distracted."

—

Daniel Goleman

The Red Queen said to Alice: "It takes all the running you can to stay in the same place." Of course, from a health perspective, this is the same woman who shouted, "Off with their heads," at the slightest provocation. Contrary to the Red Queen, by slowing down our thinking, we can actually maneuver faster and get ahead of the game. It does require us, however, to recognize the reality of where we are. Understanding and trusting the truth of this idea may be more difficult for some than they might imagine. We are suggesting something that is tough only because the very mechanism we need to change is the one that sees the problem. At the same time, we need to be willing to at least entertain the possibility that we can do more with less effort in a more reflective state. Our ability to notice the different cadences at which we operate within our own world of perception, and how each pace affects how we perceive that world, will facilitate this exploration. We need to be able to distinguish between when we are operating frenetically as opposed to operating at optimum high performance. We also need to differentiate between the numbing speed of worry and anxiety and the engaging speed of flow. Once we recognize that we do not operate at just one speed, the next step is to discover what the nature and quality of life are when we operate from health and have greater perspective and presence. Of course, we only recognize this nature and quality after the fact. But to see this at all, we have to be aware of the variable nature of our perception of reality, that is, being aware of our ever-shifting feelings, emotions, and finally, the fluctuation of our thoughts between content and process.

It is important to understand and reiterate that the process we are describing is not one that is predetermined. We can't say, today, we're going to spend the day in health or perspective or wisdom. All we can do is notice our quality of life because quality of life, as we perceive it, is an indicator of our current level of understanding or health. If we were feeling angry toward a co-worker, it would immediately indicate our health was at a low level. If, on the other hand, we were eager to remove some of the load one of our compatriots was carrying simply because we could, without any expectation, that, too, would be an indication of our current level of health.

For example, we become frustrated about something at work. Immediately, we become intolerant to stress and bad feelings, but not to the point where we actively go out and change it. We are intolerant to it so it shows up louder on our radar screens. But the moment that we realize that what we are perceiving as reality is nothing more than just a perception, we're already on the road to recovering our health. The starting point is our intolerance to those feelings. The difference between what we are suggesting here and what was "normally" considered "OK" was that a sign of our mental capacity was our ability to tolerate pressure and stress and still be functional—our "normal" setting. The more stress we could put up with and the more bad feelings we could handle, the more OK we were. We viewed this as a sign of maturity and growth. We were taught to get in touch with our dysfunction and our feelings of fear, anxiety, anticipation, or frustration so we could live with them in spite of the discomfort.

In some cases, this translated into actions such as taking skydiving lessons if we were afraid of falling. Or if we felt intimidated around authority, we put ourselves in front of authority figures. Most of us rarely see any of these choices as thought-based; as our habitual way of thinking. Instead, we see it as our responsiveness to our exterior situations.

When we take these steps, the illusion we create is that we have somehow conquered our fears, anxieties, and frustrations. But when we're confronted again by those fears and anxieties and they all return big time, we think there must be something terribly wrong with us to have failed in conquering them. Because we were unable to see the issue as our thinking in the first place, we end up simply chasing their artifacts; how they are manifested outwardly. What we create to fill the void of our understanding are our fears, frustrations, and anxieties.

Feelings, Convictions, and Beliefs

As we have mentioned, most people only recognize these issues in hindsight. There are not many who can notice their thoughts in the moment. However, one way to recognize the quality of our thinking in the moment, or as close as possible to the moment, is by the way we feel. Our sensations, emotions, and feelings are the mechanisms that enable us to realize the quality of our thinking, and they provide us with the necessary clues to avert disaster or to embrace life in its fullest. When we feel angry, enthusiastic, or humble, it is an indication of our current level of thinking. What we really are assessing here are our feelings surrounding our quality of life. Sometimes, those feelings are greater than at other times, and sometimes not. We are also trying not to categorize these moments. "Ah, there was a moment of wisdom. There was a funny moment. There was an angry moment." Once we engage in that activity, we really start missing all the moments.

It should also be mentioned that we are not asking people to forsake their strengths of conviction or beliefs. We are suggesting that we can entertain the possibility of breathing life into our often "freeze-dried" versions of truth and wisdom. Convictions and beliefs are nothing more than thoughts that have a special meaning to us. They are rules of right living or rules of how life works for us. For the most part, these thoughts embody a great deal of wisdom and have their genesis in higher thought. However, a conviction or a belief can easily become a platform for judgment that, in and of itself, indicates its artifact nature. If we can regularly access the state from which the wisdom of these convictions emerges, and let the state determine for us our course of action, then we bring to bear everything offered from that original state, including other qualities such as compassion, justice, humor, and perspective.

Convictions and beliefs are nothing more than content. We want to get past the content of thought into the process of thought, the state from which the wisdom that spawned the belief emerges. When we are dealing with content only and its associated habitual, knee-jerk reactions, our convictions become judgments. When we are in that state in which we are accessing wisdom, everything *but* judgment comes into play.

From a business perspective, we have certain convictions and beliefs that lead to ideas and rules about the way our organization needs to operate. The context here is important for our understanding.

Let us look, for instance, at the realities and myths of leadership—what we believe to be true. If we were to make a list, we might come up with things like:

- A good leader is visionary.
- A good leader is courageous.
- A good leader leads, follows, or gets out of the way.
- A good leader is results oriented.
- A good leader has perspective.
- A good leader is strategic.
- A good leader respects his or her people.

These are strong beliefs and convictions, and most leaders would undoubtedly agree these are some of the realities of leadership. However, if we were to look at these out of context, is there a time when a good leader is not results focused? Most definitely. What determines a leader's ability to make that call? Suppose a leader were to go through life saying, "Results are the only fair way to measure a person," and held that as a conviction. What happens to the culture of an organization that is driven only by results? It loses its heart and eventually finds itself in worse straights, from burnout to declining productivity and morale to sabotage, all stemming from that one conviction.

We need to tap into the wisdom from which the conviction that "results are important in the game of business—we have to turn a profit" originally arose. When we do, we also find the wisdom purporting that there are other variables we need to take into consideration. It's the state from which that initial insight arose, not the content of the insight itself, that we want to tap into. We could apply that to a belief about the bottom line, also. The greater the margin we can provide to our company's shareholders, the greater our worth. That, in and of itself, is a hard bottom-line belief. By steadfastly following that belief, we could easily drive our company and our clients crazy. That is not to say there isn't a grain of truth in that belief. But there is also a "but" in that belief, and the ability to recognize it comes from a state of wisdom.

The same thing is true with a conviction like "Teamwork is better." There is a grain of truth in that. When the truck is careening down the road out of control, it is not the time to call a caucus. There are going to be times when, as much as we want teamwork, the situation dictates that one person step forward and say, "Hey, guys, look out! We'll talk about this later, but I think if there is no real objection, we better get the hell out of the way, and we better do it now."

Once again, we want to tap into the state of wisdom out of which the initial idea surfaced, not the artifact version, which is no longer alive. In this instance, people who hold the conviction of teamwork all the time run the risk of missed opportunities because they are so busy focusing on making sure that they have the consensus of the team. This is one example of how running too fast can actually let people pass us by. What we are suggesting here is continually questioning our habitual ways of thinking. This process begins by first making those habits visible.

Learning to See Our Thoughts

We make our thought habits visible by recognizing our thoughts, but we don't stop there. If we do, we become self-conscious or end up trying to control our thoughts. When we first start making our thoughts visible, we usually only do so after the fact. But with practice, we can bring our conscious awareness closer to the moment. Then we begin noticing the quality of our life, and when we can move beyond that, we can be here now.

To illustrate this, let us draw a continuum. At the low range we would find "not seeing thought." Mid-range would be "seeing thought from a content standpoint." Top range would be "seeing what comes before thought." At the bottom would be reality: "There is no such thing as thought, I am just dealing with reality." We move up a notch and find, "Life is learning how to deal with negative emotions." We move up another notch and we come to "Life is learning my thought habits; what I do with thought." At the lower end: "There is nothing we can do with the content of our thought habits; as a matter of fact, we cannot even distinguish between content and process." We might be worriers, so we tend to worry. We might be fantasizers so we constantly live in the future. As we move up the scale of understanding, we get closer and closer to noticing the illusionary nature of thought, to the point where we go through life and are graceful with our thinking. We still do things with it, but there is no load; no excess weight to it.

Every time we notice our thoughts, we start connecting the patterns and feelings attached to those thoughts. The habitual patterns are often the ones that surface first because they are the patterns closest to our familiar feelings of life. If we were worriers, we'd notice worry. Of course, if someone asked us why we were worrying, we probably wouldn't see it as worry. We always have excellent reasons for our actions. If we were control types, we might notice when we were controlling. Again, we control for very good reasons. At some point in our memory, we deduced that controlling the situation was a good thing. We then vainly attemped to control our situations. So, we make our habitual patterns visible by first recognizing feelings that are familiar.

One of our clients described a team meeting situation with his company's CEO. In the middle of the meeting, the CEO suddenly said, "Wait a minute, I feel myself getting angry. I recognize that I am getting angry. OK, I can let go of that, let's get back to the topic." Those were his first steps toward becoming aware of his habitual patterns. Rather than blowing his fuse and blasting out at those around him, which would have been "normal," he recognized the feeling and chose to do something different. That was a choice that set in motion a whole new course of possibilities.

Slowing it down to surrender to the process of thought is tremendously healing. The CEO who recognized his anger and was able to let go of it took a mindful step. Had his response been "I wonder why I'm bothered? I wonder if anything you guys are doing bothers me?" it would lead immediately to a mind filled by the content of thought. By simply saying, "Whoa," he breathed life into the event and immediately elevated his level of understanding, as well as the understanding of those in the meeting with him. An action like that speaks volumes to all those present about how we are to conduct ourselves in an interactive situation.

It is also important to remember that as we move through this new understanding of how our thoughts affect our level of health, we needn't take ourselves too seriously. Invariably, as soon as we do, as soon as our level of self-importance overrides our healthier thoughts, our humility and our ability to laugh at ourselves evaporate and our minds fill, and that's not a funny sight.

Why Would I Ever Want to Slow It Down?

Larry Senn likens our fear of slowing it down to a juggler spinning plates on top of sticks: "We are afraid one of the plates is going to drop off the stick if we slow it down. Most people were raised to feel that 'I'm contributing more when I am doing more, thinking more, writing more.' It's the bucket of sweat syndrome. It is actually threatening to some people to have time on their hands and not to have an over-jammed schedule."

There are also some who may find it difficult to accept that slowing it down is really necessary at all. Pragmatic brains often need to see the validity for doing so. How will it make our business life less complex and more effective? What we are describing carries the sensation of slowing it down, but a slower life comes from perspective and not from our speed driving toward a goal. The pace of life is the result of our understanding, and is not determined by our consciously doing less of life. Trying to do less is impermanent, frustrating, and effortful because we are constantly focusing on doing. When life is frenetic, it is because we are frenetic. We wake up early one morning, unable to sleep, and all we can see is the workload facing us. The anxiety level rises, and we know further sleep is useless. We call this waking up outside-in. Our thoughts zoom faster, and filled agendas begin piling up before us. By the time we actually get out of bed, we're in a full-blown frenzy. Feverishly, we sit down and scratch out "to-do" notes, and as the list grows, so does our worry. Finally, a few hours later at the office, after dealing briskly with the receptionist and anyone else crossing our path, we've made a few phone calls, sent out a few e-mails, and we realize our list wasn't as impenetrable as we had conjured in bed. We feel a momentary calm.

The complexity of the world gets out-of-hand when we cannot discern between all the multiple bits of information we receive; when we can't sort between the trivial and the vital. The ability to do so comes from wisdom, insight, perspective, compassion, and common sense—all traits that occur when we are in a moment of flow rather than gripped, hectic, worried, or forced. It is also the only way we can find calm and have it last longer than a moment.

People have always gravitated toward those who can see around corners; solve our problems at a deeper, more universal level; or bring order to a seemingly chaotic world. All they have that those seeking them don't, is perspective: an ability to step back and see the larger picture for what it really is. The Wizard of Oz had no real magic behind his curtain, but he was able to see the situations of Dorothy and her friends for what they were; their habitual thinking.

That is precisely how slowing it down makes our business life less complex and more effective. It is important to restate that this notion of inner velocity may have nothing to do with the speed we might be traveling. But it does have everything to do with our ability to focus, observe, sharpen our perceptions, and be in the moment. Pace is in the eyes of the beholder. If we were to move into a world that was seemingly operating faster than we were used to, we might use pace as our reason for not enjoying it. Again, it's a matter of our perspective. There are people who can work in the stock market and not get ulcers. There is a belief that one could only work in that environment for a few years without suffering irreparable damage. But then there are also people who have made that pace their life's work without ill effect.

Similarly, as our clients experience the reality of healthy high performance, pace becomes irrelevant. The focus is on achieving the "blue chip" results; what is most important. In the hectic, mind-filled world, activity is often confused with results. The feeling is, "I'm busy. I'm active. I have a lot to do. I'm tired. I must be making progress." But as Larry Senn makes clear, the opposite is really the case: "When I quiet things down, the things that are truly the most important tend to pop up. They float to the surface and I realize that is where I need to focus. Without that reflection, everything looks important and has similar weight."

Greater perspective is the source for the answers to our issues and challenges. As groups "slow down" to hear their wisdom and common sense, the quiet can be uncomfortable as well as unfamiliar. In some cases, people complain about being bored or they need a rush of activity or a crisis to keep them going. Nonetheless, it is from our mental state of calmness (flow) that our greater answers and insights will come.

This is what the Zen master Shunryu Suzuki meant when he said, "It is easy to have calmness in inactivity. It is hard to have calmness in activity. But calmness in activity is true calmness." The pace of business is not the issue. The mindful state is.

Staying Calm When All Around You...

We might run the fastest 100 meters on record, but the only way we could find the flow to do so would be if we were totally calm and present. We see examples of the opposite situation at work all the time: people who are too tight and simply can't perform well. Some of these people may think that if they were unwound, they'd be too loose to work. They might think that to operate at their optimum state, the mechanism needs to be wound tight. This may appear to be a good thing to these people, something they thrive on, but often at the moment when peak performance is required, they can't keep up. As we have seen with athletes at moments of peril or self-defense, and with those operating successfully in the fastest of Internet industries, we perform at our best in a relaxed state. When we are in that state, we access our capabilities more quickly and appropriately as the situation demands.

When we are wound up, our minds are working furiously. We immediately step into the mind-filled world and mindfulness is lost. When this happens, any signal we send to our brain needs to be stronger because it has more thoughts to penetrate. Bruce Lee, the late martial artist extraordinaire, explained it this way: "There is only one moment of tension in fighting, 99 percent of the time you need to be completely quiet, relaxed, and in the moment. That one moment of tension is the split millisecond of contact."

What that means is that even as we are throwing a punch, we are completely relaxed. Only at the moment of contact do we tense our fist. The millisecond after that contact we return to a relaxed state. In putting this into practice, we have found that the more relaxed we are, the faster our punches become. Not only are our punches faster, but we can respond quicker to blocks. Our muscles alone simply aren't capable of that speed.

The same thing is true on a mental plane. Our brain does not have the same flexibility or responsiveness when it is stuck on one topic. An example of this would be the difference between delivering a memorized speech and being prepared, and totally in the moment and speaking extemporaneously. No matter how well-written or delivered, the memorized speech supplies little more than entertainment and polite engagement. The "in the moment" speechmaker touches people at a deeper level that stays with the audience well after the speech has been completed. Impact outweighs content.

This is why it becomes so important that at the moment of delivery, we want to be totally present. That requires mindfulness. A mind filled will miss the moment. The keys to any successful operation are relaxation, flexibility, and responsiveness. This is true in any and all business interactions, from sales to service. The more mindful we are, the better the customer's needs are addressed, because our needs are not in the way.

There are surely those who fear that any form of slowing it down only means letting the competition pass us. As we have mentioned, slowing it down mentally does not mean slowing down physically. What we are doing instead is not necessarily slowing thought, but providing some space around thought so that we are not so filled by it. That is what provides the sensation of slowing down.

So, the concern that competition might pass us by if we were to slow down is pure illusion. As a matter of fact, when operating in that state, the competition will actually (1) become more in awe of the action that we take because it will be so out of the box, and (2) feel passed by *us* because of our new, more innovative thinking and our ability to be quicker to market and responsive to our customers.

Recognizing the Quality of Life Now

The important factor in recognizing when we become too mind-filled and speeded up is being aware of the feeling surrounding our quality of life. This provides us with a clue that we are either off base or in sync with our flow. Our perception of perspective does not occur instantaneously. When we feel mind-filled, and we can recognize that hectic, over-stuffed feeling, that is our clue to perhaps give ourselves a little space, even briefly. Walk away. Sit, walk, jog, shower. Do whatever frees our mind and provides the space we need. It doesn't have to take long. We might do it automatically when we get up for a cup of coffee or take a walk through the halls of the office. Surrendering to the feeling is the first step to greater health and mindfulness.

Perhaps the first big step toward health for some may come in discovering it is OK to be intolerant of stress; to simply refuse to put up with it. Many of us have been brought up being tolerant of our stress levels, and actually try to master them. For many, society and business appear to reward and promote those individuals who can cope with the most stress and still appear functional. Work-life balance is something to be dreamt about, not lived. Rushing oneself to points of fatigue is part of the job and is sometimes treated as the professional's "red badge." When we become OK with being intolerant of stress, we can see our thinking that convinced us otherwise. We see the convictions that have made stress a good idea, that emanate from our belief that there is "good" stress, giving rise to sayings we've heard all our life like "We are on the road to laziness. Idle hands are the devil's workshop. No pain, no gain." These ideas are all memories of previous training and thought; forced mode in action.

This intolerance enables us to notice stress sooner, and the more quickly we can recognize the feeling of stress, the sooner we can step back from it rather than do battle with it. That stepping back does nothing more than allow perspective in. When we step up and battle, trying to overcome, conquer, force, or control it, we're caught by the content of the thought and our mind is quickly filled. Putting up with stress, tension, pressure, and undue obligations are what many of us consider "normal behavior." But it is not. Learning to say no to it, and stepping back, gaining perspective, and moving forward without it is "normal" and healthy behavior. And when we slow down enough to recognize that, it doesn't matter how fast the game is: We'll keep up.

Chapter Five

Experiencing Thought

"There is nothing either good or bad but thinking
makes it so."

———

William Shakespeare

We have been doing a great deal of talking about thought. In this chapter, we will provide an opportunity for the experience of thought. Following our brief introduction, we will present a series of single-page reflections that can provide us with an experience of our thought. These are only tools to provide greater insight into the process of our thinking. If confusion surfaces while you are reading through these pages, that is good.

Confusion is often a gateway to a new insight. With this understanding, confusion will not elicit insecurity or a race to clarity. From this perspective, confusion is a great state of mind. It is a state in which we can say, "I haven't thought of this in quite that way. I don't have a programmed memory-based response to that issue or situation. I can listen quietly for greater wisdom or, conversely, I can try to put something together from my past memories, prejudices, and biases." However, it is only through listening quietly that original thought can arise.

Confusion also elicits humility, and humility is the threshold to greater learning. It is our willingness to acknowledge that we don't know. It is our discomfort with this state of humility, of not knowing, that causes us to be so uncomfortable with our confusion.

There is a wide gap between being in a state of knowing and in one of not knowing. We might think that knowing would be a preferable location. After all, most of society promotes cognitive knowing as a positive way of being. Individuals who embrace this idea are often susceptible to being arrogant and judgmental. Surprisingly to some, not knowing is actually the preferable state.

The state of humility is not to be confused with meekness or self-deprecation. It is a willingness to explore, to see life completely differently, and to reinvent oneself or one's interpretation of how life works. Humility is a willingness to step away from the conventions and manifestations of success and notoriety, into a state not contingent on knowing anything. It is a state of readiness born from the moment, looking from the inside-out.

In reading the ideas that follow, we suggest allowing yourself to find a place of not knowing—a place where you are comfortable not having all the answers. In fact, while reading the ideas that follow, try not to form an answer, simply experience the thought and truly let it pass and wait for the next thought.

It is important to remember that when we come from a place of knowing the answer, arrogance arises and we no longer see humility. Arrogance is about being better than someone else. Humility, however, is not seeing ourselves as smaller or lesser. It is a state of seeing the grandeur of life and the role we play in it.

When reading what follows, allow yourself to let your thoughts flow. Whatever thought comes to you, try not to hold onto it. What you will find is that the real value of any insight that might emerge is not in its content, but in your ability to simply have the insight. What you're trying to release here is judgment. It surfaces quickly. When it does, realize that it, too, is a thought that can be let go so that new thoughts can enter in. The key, as well, is to not become judgmental about your judgments. This allows you to also develop a gentleness with yourself that eventually translates to the manner in which you treat others.

Society is the relationship between you and me;
and if our relationship is based on ambition, each
one of us wanting to be more powerful than the
other, then obviously we shall always be in conflict.

—

J. Krishnamurti

If ambition is to assist us in some way, how can we accomplish this from a "higher state"? What is the "higher" state?

Not knowing, that is, being willing to admit that we don't know, is one of the keys that opens the door to creative intelligence. It takes humility to open that door. Our ego doesn't like not knowing and would prefer to go over and over what we already think and believe rather than trust in a subtle, unknown process like creative intelligence.

—

Richard Carlson and Joseph Bailey

How do you know when your ego is defending itself? When is it not?

The way of cowardice is to embed ourselves in
a cocoon, in which we perpetuate our habitual
patterns. When we are constantly recreating our
basic patterns of behavior and thought, we never
have to leap into fresh air or onto fresh ground.

—

Chögyam Trungpa

Can you tell the difference between doing things differently, doing different things, and seeing life differently? If so,
what's the difference? How are they similar?

Just sheer life cannot be said to have a purpose,
because look at all the different purposes it has all
over the place. But each incarnation, you might
say, has a potentiality, and the mission of life is to
live that potentiality. How do you do it? My
answer is, "Follow your bliss." There's something
inside you that knows when you're in the center,
that knows when you're on the beam or off the
beam.

—

Joseph Campbell

What is "your bliss"? How can you tell?

The negative effects of thought arise when we lose sight of thought recognition—when we forget that we are thinking and that our thinking is creating our experience.

—

Richard Carlson and Joseph Bailey

What's the difference between being aware of your thinking and being self-conscious? (How effective are you and how do you feel when you are self-conscious?)

I learned early that one of the most important
qualities of a leader is listening without judgment,
or with what Buddhists call *bare attention.*

—

Phil Jackson

The very mechanism you use to notice when you are not
in "bare attention" seems to be the very mechanism you want
to avoid. Can you cause yourself to be in this state? When
you are aware of this, is this "bare attention"? How can you be
there more of the time?

Nothing can bring you peace but yourself.

—

Ralph Waldo Emerson

What kind of peace do you bring to yourself?

The only Zen you find on the tops of mountains is
the Zen you bring up there.

—

Robert M. Pirsig

How do you bring Zen to the mountaintop?

You need to start trusting yourself enough to know that when you need an answer or an idea, quieting your mind—instead of filling it with data—may provide the best possible answer or solution.

—

Richard Carlson

In doing this, how does one come upon the "best" possible answer or solution? Why?

…where there is fear there is no intelligence…. To live is to find out for yourself what is true, and you can do this only when there is freedom, when there is continuous revolution inwardly, within yourself.

—

J. Krishnamurti

How would you do this? What role does your thinking play? As you define "reality," what influence does it have on your fear level?

Our thinking creates problems that the same level
of thinking can't solve.

—

Albert Einstein

How do you know if you've "solved" the problem?

Experience without theory teaches us nothing.

—

W. Edward Deming

What does this mean? How many interpretations can you come up with?

Linear thinking, grand strategy thinking, formulaic thinking, conventional thinking, credentialed thinking, produce only comforting illusions, bland rigidities, complacent passivity, all the slow-working recipes for disaster.

—

James Champy

If this is true, what is the antidote? What does one need to avoid the results of this paragraph?

Always leave enough time in your life to do
something that makes you happy, satisfied, or even
joyous. That has more of an effect on economic
well-being than any other single factor.

—

Paul Hawken

How is this true? How does doing something that makes
you happy, satisfied, or joyous impact your economic well-
being?

You've got to be very careful if you don't know
where you are going, because you might not
get there.

—

Yogi Berra

How many dimensions of "there" does your life embrace?
What are they?

Chapter Six

Mindful Leadership

"Strategy is important. But once you've done the mental work, there comes a point when you have to throw yourself into the action and put your heart on the line. That means not only being brave, but also being compassionate toward yourself, your teammates, and your opponents."

—

Phil Jackson

We mandate our leaders with the explicit permission to do what it takes to achieve healthy profitability, results, growth, competitiveness, image, and brand, and to change and recharge any of these issues should they flag. What we find, however, is that there is a great deal of disparity between what is considered healthy and what is not. Some leaders believe their charter allows them to pursue profitability, results, and growth at all costs as long as the bottom line increases year after year in upward spirals of exponential degrees that meet analysts' expectations. This "Damn the torpedoes, full-speed ahead" approach may play well in movies, but movies only last a couple of hours. Quarterly reports aside, leaders who want their businesses to remain healthy for the long term need to focus further ahead

The height of mind-filled leadership, often driven by the quarterly report, would be that which is locked and loaded in reaction mode with no space for the forward and peripheral vision required by leadership. While this web-speed market place has forced many organizations to maintain a tight and vigilant focus on their enterprises, leaders who get stuck in the minutia-filled mindset of micro-management are not leading their organizations, but operating them. Out of this context, we would like to offer two different leadership perspectives that are both trying to sustain evolution, growth, and change in our organizations—one process-oriented and the other more mechanical in nature.

Leaders who see organizations from a more mechanical perspective are often those who believe they can and must drive the business hard because, after all, it is a mechanical operation that needs to be driven. However, without constant attention, mechanisms have a tendency to break, or at the very best, degrade with wear. When change is required, mechanical leadership believes it can simply attach changes onto the existing works, making the quick fix. Unfortunately, this approach only creates more effort and stress on the mechanism by constantly forcing an inherently non-flexible apparatus to adjust on the fly. Invariably, these external changes are short-lived. Not only don't they address the real problems that exist within organizations, but in their brevity, they, in turn, create high levels of cynicism within the people of the organization who don't, and often can't, see change and adaptation as part and parcel of their duties. In addition, the mechanistic leader frequently doesn't see that by applying these external patches, all he or she is doing is masking the problem and only temporarily restraining the stress that created the breakdown in the first place. What the leader is missing, of course, is that organizations are not machines but living, cultural entities that need to be treated as such. When this is ignored, the business eventually loses its life force, the very capacity that helped it reach whatever success it may have found.

In contrast, a leader who views his or her enterprise from a process perspective is more apt to take into account the cyclical nature of life that recognizes and allows for growth and regeneration. This approach doesn't require all the constant care and effort of the mechanical perspective because it operates in accordance with the natural process of adaptability and flexibility, which creates integrated and aligned change. It also frees the leader from a finely focused operational perspective, allowing a far more healthy perspective for both the organization and the leader, which is broader in nature and able to see what is new and forward moving. This perspective not only takes into account the health of an organization's results and profitability, but also doesn't lose sight that, at heart, it's a living, breathing entity full of potential and capacity.

When leaders operate from a healthy state, they understand the need for balance, and that profitability and health go hand-in-hand. As Atmos Energy's Best describes it, "I view leadership as being a servant of the people. The higher you go, the more you become a servant of the people. Lincoln said it: 'Let me see where the people are so that I can get out in front of them.' I think that 98 percent of the time that is true. Many leaders' attitudes are, 'I'm going to be successful and you can come or not; I don't care.' They don't treat their people as a valuable commodity. It is not pay and benefits that motivate people. It's environment. It's appreciation. It's being involved in something that they know they can influence."

In contrast, the more mechanical, mind-filled approach is to blindly pursue profitability and growth at the expense of the health of the people, and ultimately, the organization. At times, in a more subtle fashion and for the sake of saving a few dollars, clarifying, inspiring, or energizing events are minimized or eliminated.

We see this in failed mergers continually. When the health of the combined cultures is poor and not addressed, like any living organism, it will ultimately die. In the meantime, this new conglomerate entity will never perform to its true and healthy potential.

When leaders' states of mind are solely focused on profitability and the bottom line, and they enter into a merger to access economy of scale or more markets, it may all make sense on paper, but what is ignored is that which is going to make the merger happen: the health of the people.

The Leadership Dimension

Intuitively, leaders understand that long-term and evolving performance is directly related to the healthy state of mind of their people. However, many leaders also believe that they can cause the state of mind of others to become healthier. Now, at one level, this may appear to be the case, that external forces and situations can cause people to enter this high-performance state. Again, with all the right intentions to accomplish this, we put a great deal of effort and energy into the creation of team agreements, vision statements, and behavioral descriptions of core operating values. We conduct events intended to excite and rally our people.

In taking these steps, we require others to act in a caring way, to treat others with respect, to be creative and accountable, and to work as a team. In and of itself, these are worthy endeavors if conducted in a healthy state of mind. However, sometimes our goals get ahead of our intention.

We have entered into situations in which relationships have been seriously injured in attempting to come up with a definition of teamwork. We have seen teams so fatigued from their journey to define their vision that they need a vacation from the words. And, in a few situations, we have encountered employees who feel battered and threatened by how the company's core values are used as a "club" against them.

We have found that the basic assumption that the psychological and spiritual health of people directly affects their effectiveness in life is true. The better our state of mind, the better we feel and the better we perform. However, for the past 20 years, after working with various leaders in business, in the community, and in government, we have found that the long-term answer does not come in the form of systems, procedures, or structure, nor is it inherently embodied in team exercises or behavioral techniques. This is an outside-in approach.

The continuous journey of increasing personal well-being and perspective is actually an inside-out phenomenon. The more that we try to force or cause others to act or feel a certain way, the further we move them away from this understanding. We inadvertently convince them that forces outside of themselves cause how they feel about themselves or a given situation. When we try to convince them of their accountability—the best that we can hope to accomplish in this scenario—the outcome always carries the feeling of blame, obligation, inadequacy, or guilt.

Those of us who are parents become especially aware of this. If one of our children does something inappropriate, we often require them to apologize or make amends. "But I don't feel sorry nor do I feel like it was my fault," comes the child's response. Because of our lack of awareness, our only recourse is to get them to at least *behave* or *act* like they are repentant. To do this, we try to convince them what the "right" thing to do is, and that it speaks to their character. If that doesn't work, we might go in another direction, using guilt, remorse, or fear of punishment to get them to act accordingly. We, of course, do not have an answer to their next question "… but Dad, if I do that, isn't that lying?"

How often do we take this approach with the people we lead? What if we don't feel respectful of others and it's a core value? What if we feel victimized or taken advantage of by our company or boss, and personal accountability is the stated pillar of the company? What if we don't feel heard, and effective listening is one of the team's agreements? What if we're afraid to make a mistake, and risk-taking is a required dimension of performance? What if we don't feel inspired and we have to share the vision with other employees or with our customers? What do we do?

Until we understand that how our children feel is a function of how they think, we are powerless when they feel angry or put upon. We don't know how to raise the health of their thinking. Unfortunately, out of ignorance, we often drive them deeper into their helpless state. The same, of course, is true with those with whom we work.

For many of us, both at home and in business, this is the best we can do. We've read and researched the "best practices" on how leaders should act, but we don't have the eyes to see the tremendous potency in raising our states of mind, improving our perspectives, and increasing our psychological health. As Larry Senn explains, "In less healthy organizations, the leader is often part of the problem rather than the solution to the problem. The healthier leaders believe that one of the greatest resources they have is the health of their organization. They are very respectful of that, and if they see it going sideways, they intervene. They see that leading the attitudes, behaviors, and culture is as important as leading the strategy."

Bob Gunn concurs: "The most important thing for me is to foster my own innate health and to show up that way. I think that is 90 percent of it. The other component is to be a point of continuous direction for people. As the leader, it is incumbent upon me to really be in sync with that vision and be a living example, keeping it alive and in front of people."

Imagine the tremendous service leaders could provide if they could enable this in themselves as well as in others? Imagine being able to weatherproof ourselves from the hardships of business? Imagine the resiliency and performance of businesses that come from their people being able to maintain their bearings as well as to continually see and implement creative ways to ensure the success of their company. In many ways, the most important dimension for leaders to learn revolves around being aware of the quality of their own thinking and enabling the people with whom they work to bring out their best efforts more of the time.

Developing New Leaders

Strategically, our ability to recognize this dimension comes at a most opportune time. The organization of the future needs to enable more and more "leaders" to emerge. No longer can successful companies survive and prosper under the guidance of one or two determining leaders while the rest of the organization operates as dutiful followers or merely competent implementers. The evolution of business seems to indicate that more "virtual" leaders are needed in the grand scheme as challenges, objectives, and operational dimensions change.

Every company in today's market place is dealing with rapidly changing business scenarios, increasing competition, more complex people issues, more demanding and sophisticated clients, opportunities and challenges of technology, and an ever-evolving global economy. Regardless of the situation or their approach to leadership, each corporate leader with whom we have worked has three goals on his/her mind:

1. How can I make my company even more competitive and successful as well as guarantee its future?

2. How can I better serve all my stakeholders?

3. How can I raise the morale, teamwork, openness, effectiveness, and well-being of the people working for my company?

Healthy High-performance Leadership

To achieve these goals, our leaders must operate and function optimally, which hinges on their ability to be in an optimal state of mind. This healthy, high-performance state is what we have called mindfulness. As we have mentioned, we cannot will this state into existence, no matter what our position in an organization might be, and we only notice it after the fact. How then do we achieve this state of *healthy* high performance? And, how do leaders bring this state into their organization? Not surprisingly, the answer comes from principles we find all around us.

What follows then should raise some questions as to how well we access this healthy high-performance state for ourselves, and how well we do this for others.

- *Respect and Appreciate Our State of Health*: If anything, much of what we have been doing in business has emanated from the basic assumption that there is a healthy, high-performance state of being. However, once we have visited this state, we often attempt to capture it in behavioral statements—dos and don'ts of correct action—and then tie them down with mutual team agreements. Just look at our vision statements, which are meant to inspire and capture the creativity and accountability of employees and give hope and meaning to our clients, suppliers, and partners. Or our values statements, which are descriptions of what we think healthy high-performance looks like in our company. Even when we talk about leadership, teamwork, coaching, accountability, and support, we translate these healthy states into rigid descriptions of behavior. Too often, after these statements are distributed, we are asked to bring the spirit back into the statements around which we mold the organization.

We are suggesting that beyond the behavioral statements is a state of mind that enables and empowers people to act in an appropriate way in all situations. Instead of "freeze-drying" this healthy state, we recommend that we notice in ourselves the feeling of being in this state and understand some of the dynamics affecting it.

- *Gently Notice When I'm Not There*: Considering the fact that we cannot tell when we are in the "zone" while we are in it, the next best thing is to notice when we are not there. This, in and of itself, is an interesting exploration since it manifests itself in myriad ways.

   What are our clues? For some it's a feeling of insecurity, anger, or tension. When this happens, do we wait for these feelings to pass before taking action; or do we jump into these feelings, express our anger, look for reasons why we feel this way; or look into our history to see if this could be a condition of our character? If we wait for a moment, we will notice ourselves regaining perspective that will enable us to handle the situation much more effectively and with greater security. We are not ignoring problems, but instead, handling them in the best way we are capable of doing.

Regardless of what it is for each of us, this state of mind will make the world and all in it appear to justify why we feel the way we do. If we can merely see it as our thinking and that our thoughts are of our own doing, we will be able to step onto the path of self-healing and subsequently more effectively deal with the situation. Simply realize that our health will naturally ebb and flow. At one moment we may feel low, and the very next, we might be at the top of our game.

Although we are always thinking, the quality of the experience and the quality of the thoughts themselves vary from moment to moment. It's the "quiet mind" that leads to this healthy high-performance state. Remember, we can appear to be very active and still be in this "zone" of quiet health and awareness. By understanding this, we can be much more graceful around the twists and turns of life.

- *Do I See People as Basically "Good"*?...or do I see them as basically flawed, damaged goods? Again, many of us might become aware of this issue via an example at home.

  We might be staunch disciplinarians who truly believe that every deep lesson has to be learned with appropriate remorse or guilt. Many men we've spoken with will watch their wives work with their children and honestly feel she's way too soft with them, allowing them to get away with "murder." These fathers then, in an attempt to avoid raising potentially "spoiled criminals," skillfully browbeat their adolescents until a tear of remorse or guilt is shed.

One afternoon after one of these sessions involving one of the authors, his wife turned to him and asked, "Honey, how do you see our kids? Do you see them as basically good and loving individuals only needing our direction, love, and an occasional firm hand, or do you see them as basically bad, needing us to teach them right from wrong?" After a few agonizing moments of self-reflection, he realized that because of his own insecurity and conditioned thinking, he could not see the "goodness" and "capabilities" that already resided in his children. He realized the resulting stance he took determined how he dealt with his children...and with everyone else in his life. His overly cautious, lack of trust was a direct result of this stance. His quickness to judge others or see their actions as emanating from self-serving motives stood in the way of working effectively with others, especially in trying or challenging times. He found himself talking down to people or arrogantly trying to teach them the right way of living or attending to business. And after all of this effort, very little was accomplished, other than to drive them further away.

The realization that came from this awareness was that people are attracted to those who tend to bring out the best in them. They are more inspired, accountable, and forward moving under this assumption. They are more accepting of the reality of the situation and less likely to get frightened by different situations. They start to see their innate strength, wisdom, and goodness for themselves, and act accordingly. Even though they may not address issues in the same manner that we would, performance improves and problems get solved.

- *Humility is the Doorway to Continuous Learning and Improvement:* From an early age, we have been taught that always knowing the answer is desirable. We become uneasy with the state of "not knowing" or humility. Sometimes this is taken to a point where having an opinion, regardless of whether it is right or wrong, is better than not having any opinion at all. Our willingness to wait for an answer is diminished as we rush to conclusions. Our intolerance with perceived failure is directly related to our discomfort with humility. As such, we often limit our learning to intellectual lessons that reinforce our preexisting level of awareness, thus preventing real breakthroughs and shifts in paradigm. Our discomfort causes us to avoid responsible risk-taking and to stick with the straight and narrow path. We hesitate to offer new ideas in the face of possibly being wrong or looking foolish in others' eyes. But remember, our foolishness only looks that way to those who also have difficulty with humility.

Executives that sustain change and growth within themselves and in their organizations understand and respect humility. These leaders frequently build on what they know, and willingly explore new ways of doing business. It's important to note that humility, certainty, and confidence are all cut from the same cloth. Humility is a very responsive state of mind— one that is open to new lessons, and at the same time, not hesitant to act on what is seen.

Humility is an open stance toward life—curious, appreciative, and humbled by its potential. These individuals realize that it doesn't really matter how "big or small" we are when measured against others, but that humility comes from appreciating and being in awe with how wondrously "big" life is.

Business leaders who seem to keep pushing the edge of the envelope understand this state of mind. They appear to do this regardless of how business is doing. For many, it makes sense to explore change when business is bad. But the leader who understands this stance will do the same thing when things are going well.

- *Forgiveness is the Key to Moving Forward*: Every now and then, we have in our programs two teammates who have been at odds with one another for a number of years. Their feuds and off-handed comments have become legendary in the culture of the company.

  These difficulties melt away when these individuals can see the role that their thoughts play in defining their reality of the situation. They also notice the arbitrary and neutral nature of these thoughts and how much of their attitude was based on old memories. They see how much of their "reality" was created from their own imagination filling in the blanks. When they become aware of their thinking in a healthy way, they gain greater perspective and have the capacity to move forward from a fresh start.

More than once, we have witnessed that when these two antagonists see the innocence in their own thinking as well as in the thinking of their perceived adversary, years of ill feelings appear to fall by the wayside, and they start their relationship afresh. Frequently, they can laugh at their past incursions and they never seem to return to those "bad" days again. Through forgiveness, they experience an insight that changes how they see life, themselves, and each other, forever.

Show us an organization in which forgiveness is not a vital part of the culture, and we will show you an organization afraid to take risks or think outside of the box. Forgiveness is a healthy state of mind that sees the innocence in the way people think and the subsequent link with their actions. The state of forgiveness does not mean that all actions are arbitrarily condoned, ignored, or approved. It does mean, though, that appropriate corrections, learning, and actions are taken without recrimination, resentment, or revenge. Through forgiveness, there is a keen sense of perspective, timeliness, and wisdom that shines through the behaviors and the decisions.

Without forgiveness, there can be no change of heart. Without a change of heart, we are condemned to carry around others as well as our own mistakes and shortcomings every day of our lives. A change of heart allows us to start anew with every moment. As a very wise mentor once told us, "Individuals without forgiveness are like computers without delete keys—the screen continues to fill up with mistakes leaving very little room for productive work."

- *Listening = 80 Percent of the Time*: Effective leaders and teammates with whom we have worked have been excellent listeners. They are present in the moment with the other person and can listen beyond the content of the conversation. They can "sense" feelings, are profoundly curious, and "hear" subtleties that escape even the speaker. Through listening, they bring healing to the situation and raise the conversation to a level in which solutions and possibilities can be explored.

  Unfortunately, this is not the norm for most people. We have been taught that to be a leader means that you are the one who does the influencing. Many people then extrapolate that stance and direct it toward listening. When they listen, they do so to strengthen their ability to influence others. They define influence as always having to have the answers as well as pressing those answers upon others. When impatience or judgments set in, these leaders interrupt and provide the answers. Regardless of the situation, they frequently assume that they know the full issue. When this happens, the issue is rarely truly resolved, and much to the chagrin of all involved, will need to be addressed a second or third time.

We have found that healthy leaders appear so confident in their security and personal well-being that they listen to be truly influenced by what the speaker is saying. They do not arbitrarily accept everything that is shared with them. Rather, they learn to listen for the "grains of truth" and the points of common sense in the speaker's thinking. They listen to be "touched" as well as to satisfy their tremendous curiosity. They have respect and good will for the speaker throughout the exchange. Only by fully experiencing the world of the speaker can the listener respond accurately and appropriately. This is true for any relationship whether in management or sales, while negotiating, or in parenting and marriage.

A more subtle result of effective and deep listening is the leader's ability to learn, internalize, and apply new information and ideas. The majority of time, we hear about the brilliance and quickness of leaders. They seem to be able to quickly integrate new approaches, technology, and strategies in their own behaviors and approaches to the business. We have found that their ability to listen to the point where their own ideas are changeable, yet not threatened, is a characteristic that few people possess. Most have learned to defend their thinking rather than listen for grains of truth, common sense, or wisdom coming from others. They see influencing others as meaning not being influenced themselves. Nothing could be farther from the truth.

The questions arise: Am I known for my ability to bring out the best in others or only for my own ingenious and creative problem solving? And, commensurately, am I known for my listening ability? Do people truly feel heard by me? Do people feel that I am a difficult person to introduce new ideas to or that I too often play the role of "devil's advocate" or obstructionist? Am I known for my ability to take an idea, identify the "grains of truth," and with others, build on them? Am I known to be a "quick study" or one who can grasp the subtle nuances of a situation or idea? Do people feel better after a conversation with me regardless of whether or not their proposal was accepted? It's easy to notice how closely linked these dimensions are to one another. We have found that asking these questions to those around us provides some very interesting feedback as well.

- *It's an Inside-Out Life.* Volumes have been written about a transcendent state of mind that extends beyond the obvious and taps into both a higher and deeper level of wisdom and rapport. We have noticed that those leaders who see themselves as a conduit to this wisdom seem to do the best, appear to be able to anticipate issues, maintain their bearings the easiest, and can speak to the hearts of their people. They have a well-developed sense of service to their company and its clients, and to the community. But, at a deeper level, they can differentiate the quality of their thoughts to discern what we call transcendent thought from personal thought, or insight from strategy. They have become adept at noticing and following transcendent thought more of the time. But behind this capacity is their acceptance that transcendent thought exists and that its source is beyond memory, analysis, or past experiences. Through this understanding and seeing, a visionary leader can stand apart from others but not stand alone. They appear weatherproofed from life's challenges and enjoy everything that life has to offer, not just the good.

Regardless of what name these leaders attach to this transcendent source, they all seem to share these common traits and characteristics. Because of their keen sense of integrity, conscience, and character, others around them feel confident that they will be given a fair shake. Their boundless stance of being in service seems to be endless and ever-changing. Some are religious and some are not, but they all seem to possess tremendous perspective on the moment and rarely, if ever, lose their bearings. Finally, they all seem to play to a more distant horizon, but will do whatever is necessary and appropriate in the moment.

Once we can recognize this state of leadership within ourselves, we can then begin to more clearly see how it manifests itself in the workplace. We find, for instance, that the way in which a leader crafts and implements the culture and values of an organization is based on his or her own self-knowledge and grounding. Those values that seem most alive to a leader are those with which the leader is most directly grounded. Secondly, he or she must be able to turn what is an intellectually good idea into a personal awareness of how they see life. This is important because the subtle (and/or not so subtle) modeling of a leader provides instinctive information about the leader's commitment to these ideas to both the senior team and the organization.

This is why it is imperative that the values of the culture be developed from within the same state of mind that these values are intended to elicit and describe. The source of such thinking, of course, is mindfulness. In coming from this state of mind, the leader allows these vision and value statements to evolve naturally. It is also up to the leader to minimize the amount of word-smithing to keep people more in a flow state than in one of judgment, evaluation, comparison, and analysis.

Often one of the biggest problems we encounter is a content-correct vision and value statement that is incapable of moving anyone in any direction. This usually happens when those developing these ideas have a moment of inspiration and put the ideas on paper, but instead of staying in that state of inspiration, they move into a state of analysis. Since the vision and values of an organization are meant to enable people to tap into the same inspiration and creativity out of which they were formed, it makes sense that these statements should be crafted from within the state of mind they are meant to draw out. Unfortunately, in many cases, these ideas are communicated from a purely content and intellectual standpoint, and the carefully crafted words never come alive.

The state of leadership out of which the leader operates also enables or disables the health of the organization. This is manifested in the way the leader

- models health,
- accesses higher states of mind to solve problems and provide solutions,
- exhibits his or her grounding in these ideas,
- creates a presence in the organization,
- understands the form and formlessness of process, and recognizes that listening is his or her primary communication device.

Seldom do we think of listening as a communication device, let alone one that is primary. As we mentioned earlier, it is a powerful tool for communicating our presence and intent, as well as a means for accessing wisdom. But beyond that, what we find is that people who live extremely healthy lives have an impact on others purely by the example they provide. A mindful leader can accelerate that impact by translating his or her understanding and grounding, and then articulating and modeling the concepts of health so that others in the organization are influenced and touched by them.

A good example of this is the way in which a leader might differentiate between coaching, feedback, and judgment. If there is no love in a leader's heart when providing coaching or feedback, then, inevitably, all they deliver to others is judgment. Judgment is a state of personal unacceptability. True coaching comes from a state of caring and accepting of the humanity of others. This does not mean that someone's unhealthiness is to be accepted, pardoned or ignored. If non-judgmental coaching doesn't lead a person toward health, the mindful leader may simply have to recognize that person may not be in the right work environment.

In large organizations, a leader's physical presence is often limited, so it is important that the leader also understands the form and formlessness of his or her influence. The form of influence is fairly easy to grasp. It takes the shape of such things as policies and procedures, as well as communication and strategy programs. The formless aspects of influence include giving people the permission to perform in a flow state as opposed to applying a curriculum or set of policies to direct and/or limit their process.

By doing this, the mindful leader is really encouraging and activating the distributed intelligence of the work force. This is an innately common sense thing to do, but it is often a step that leaders fear rather than embrace. However, by accessing the distributed intelligence of the organization— the knowledge that exists in every individual in the organiza-tion—the leader and executive team no longer have to con-cern themselves with the myriad ways that influence takes place. They can instead focus on the distractions, mindsets, and insecurities that limit communication. To do this, the mindful leader will have to let go of his or her own control-ling issues that may serve as obstacles.

We see today, more than ever, examples of leaders who keep their organizations informed about the state of the busi-ness and the strategies the organization plans to pursue. In doing so, they solicit and then mine the collective wisdom and intelligence of the entire organization. Xerox PARC's John Seely Brown, Director of Xerox's research division, believes that real innovation and new ideas come from the peripheries of an organization and not from its central core. It is at the peripheries that organizations interface in a direct fashion with the world at large. When an organization encourages and mines the distributed intelligence of those operating at the edges of its business, it brings forth new and different perspectives that are often hidden from those operating within the central core.

But more than the form of being on the periphery, the mindful leader needs to look at the mindsets and thinking patterns of the people there. The reality is that being on the periphery actually has very little to do with innovation and new ideas. The fact that this is a source for new ideas probably has more to do with a perspective not clouded by the core views. These people have an almost tacit permission to think differently because they are experiencing less control from the core. The mindful person, however, is aware that permission to be innovative and think creatively is innate in us all. Imagine if everyone in the company lived and implemented the wisdom and grains of truth inherent in most procedures and were willing to advocate change based on common sense. Positive evolution would be an ongoing way of life.

If we return to the two styles of leadership with which this chapter began, the mechanical and the process-led, the limitations of the mechanical perspective in this current business climate should be much more obvious. There was a time when this may not have been the case, when business was more predictable and manufacturing processes tolerated a more mechanistic point of view. But leadership today must contend with a far more complex and rapidly evolving landscape. Rigid systems will no longer carry the day. Our leaders are recognizing that they can't be the lone leader at the top, solely empowered to make all the decisions necessary to run an organization. As soon as we move into a more relationship-dependent model in which the interaction of teams and teams of teams are required to keep our businesses functioning smoothly, we must become more conscious of the health and organic nature of those interactions.

At the heart of this process is the health of the leader. Regardless of the situation, the leader's health will determine the eventual outcome of the organization. Many recurring problems and situations that businesses face arise because there is no clear understanding of this phenomenon, and they are destined to repeat these failings until they learn this lesson. The good news is that, as we have heard from those quoted in this chapter, there are leaders out there who do understand this relationship, and their organizations are healthier and more prosperous because of it.

Chapter Seven

Aligned Interactions

"When we are afraid of ourselves and afraid of the seeming threat the world presents, then we become extremely selfish. We want to build our own little nests, our own cocoons, so that we can live by ourselves in a secure way...Fundamentally, there is nothing that either threatens or promotes our point of view. The four seasons occur free from anyone's demand or vote. Hope and fear cannot alter the seasons."

—

Chögyam Trungpa

Everything in nature is relationship, from the quarks in an atom to organizations within industries to the planets in the solar system. Although there may be an illusion of uniqueness, nothing stands alone. Perhaps the greatest successes come from those individuals who can see this and best foster their connection. As physics has shown us, the potential for everything we have done, created, or invented has always been there. It's just been dormant waiting for our ability to catch up to its potential. To use an example from the physical world, when the planet Pluto was discovered by Clyde

Tombaugh in 1930, it wasn't a matter of the planet being newly created. It was always there. It was up to astronomers to figure that it might exist, and then up to Tombaugh to find it. The fact that we did not discover it until the twentieth century did not negate the fact that it was always there. The same is true of our innate potential for health and those things that keep us from that innate state.

With active relationships as a given in nature, it is interesting that traditionally in business we have tended to sectionalize how our organizations are run. We sectionalize into different departments, divisions, corporations, and industries, all of which, as a consequence, are separated from the environmental world.

If we were to take a look at some of the most innovative advances made in recent years, they would come from those people who are blind to those arbitrary walls. We are increasingly seeing unique relationships and partnerships occurring in the corporate world. Silos are coming down and departments are talking to one another. Those leaders who can continue breaking down these boundaries and can establish creative partnerships will be the ones who will get the jump on the competition. Those who create more effective and healthy relationships within their organizations are going to get more done, too. Aligned interactions are the true power base of the Mindful Corporation.

As business life moves more quickly, people who live segmented, structured lives and don't see that the segmentation is of their own making are going to discover they are living at a disadvantage.

This has a great deal to do with our reluctance to accept

that as humans we have no objective perspective. It all looks so real, but all we really have is a subjective reality of the world. We still feel a dimension of objective reality: We can touch a table, drive a car, and prepare and eat food, but our experience of objective reality is based purely on our subjective influence. Since our subjective perception is really all we have, it is difficult to be fully conscious of it or its impact on the way life presents itself. For example, a recent study that has dismayed pharmaceutical companies has suggested that some placebos are proving as effective in dealing with medical problems than the drugs designed to do so.

This should come as no surprise. The German physicist Werner Heisenberg (1901-1976) noted in his Principle of Uncertainty that the perceiver perceiving is always affecting what is perceived. This extends to our health in all areas of life; perspective shapes perception, which, in turn, shapes what is seen.

We have found that the amount of perspective a person has is a function of psychological and spiritual distance. Psychologically, we're referring to our ability to step back from the content of our thinking so we can see where we become stuck in our habitual patterns of thought. Before we define what we mean by spiritual distance, we should mention that the derivation of the word spirit comes from the root "to give breath to"—to breathe life into. Spiritual distance in this instance is the space between what we make most real and our perception of it. The degree to which we can slow down, as we discussed earlier, and spend time in the unfilled space of our minds is the degree to which we can gain an increasing perspective. When we are mindful, we see clearly that thought is the conduit between the object of reality and our subjective perception.

To build healthy relationships, we must understand that what is real for us is *only* real for us. To establish and maintain these relationships, we must learn to cultivate and integrate our ability to grow rapport and good will with others. We do this by raising our understanding of how our mind, consciousness, and thinking affect every interaction we have. Interestingly, it only takes one person to start this journey. There is a misconception that rapport takes two. It does not. If we come from a place of compassion and understanding, rapport automatically makes our relationships different.

Coming From Rapport

Rapport is a state of mind. Most people think of rapport as an activity or a result. Coercion is also a state of mind. The state of rapport enables us to work with others with the least resistance. This is the foundation for effective listening. If we find a person in the state of rapport, in short order we see and feel the influence of it on our relationship. Ron Adams describes this effect in relation to his former boss, Bob Best. "Bob has a tremendous gift for rapport. We could be discussing something with which I am not in alignment, and it comes to a point where Bob says, 'Listen, we've been around the barn a couple of times, we aren't going to resolve it. This is the direction we are going to go. As your leader, I have to go this direction, and get in line with me.' Because of that rapport, I'm aligned."

At the very least, we see the influence rapport has on our

ability to hear things at a deeper level. A person's ability to respond in an appropriate fashion is actually heightened because he is in a state of rapport.

This brings up a recent development that is of particular concern in today's virtual companies: The need to come from a state of rapport takes on an even greater significance when there is physical separation between people. On one level, this can have a tremendous amount of negative potential when neglected. If we get to the point in our organization where we only communicate via e-mail, we are locking ourselves into purely content-driven relationships. We lose everything from inflection and visual signals to laughter; all the subtleties of communication are stripped away. The mindful approach will be particularly important as our dependence on this form of communication increases.

A Continuum of Relationships

This is just one reason why it is so important to foster the idea of aligned interactions within a Mindful Corporation. Again, we are speaking about relationships and the characteristics of that state of relating. What follows here is a look at relationships within three different scenarios. There are undoubtedly more ways of relating than these three, but by way of example, they will serve our purposes.

These three scenarios range from the low end of the spectrum, in which we find relationships that are highly stressful and effortful, to those at the high end where relationships are more effortless and graceful. In the "healthier" scenario, decisions are made more easily and are supported by everyone involved. Conflicting situations are resolved with creative solutions that satisfy all parties. Relationships are bolstered and strengthened.

We have run into a number of situations that appear to embrace our first scenario of the adversarial mindset, culture, and leader. At this level of relating, the skill required to make things happen is the ability to debate or argue well—to be able to stand in and battle back in times of adversity. It is an exercise in applying power, authority, and influence. It can also be played out physically through intimidation and threats. We find initial implications of adversarial environments through the imposed use of titles and credentials. As an outcome of this exercise in power, adversarial relating is very stressful and takes a tremendous amount of effort to get anything accomplished. Often, in adversarial organizations, the primary determining factors are the two "f"s: fear and fatigue. People often run out of steam in a relational exchange and lose the will to fight back. "All right, you win," is the exhausted call. With that simple utterance, we have created a win-lose scenario, driven by the illusion of short-term gain and the reality of long-term pain. In a mind-filled organization like this, there is little or no collaboration and virtually no active listening, except the listening that takes place to bolster and strengthen one's position.

There are many people who see life this way. They can be charming on the surface, but only to make their point, and the next second they can be our worst nightmare. An organization like this is a highly manipulative environment. Once we become aware of this organizational mindset, it becomes obvious in relationships throughout the company.

The next level is what most organizations hope to achieve.

It is the win-win level, that place where we find a state of agreement. The adversarial level was about debate. This state is about negotiation and compromise. Often at this level, people feel they have to give up something in order to gain something. There is little building on whatever grains of truth might be in other people's points of view. At this level of awareness, we are simply trying to make the grains of truth that we know work. As might be expected, this state takes a good deal of effort, but not as much as the adversarial state does, nor is it as painful. It appears to work because there is a feeling of win-win. At the very least, however, it is a watering down of people's positions, which requires effort not only to achieve a level of agreement, but to maintain it.

Suppose, for example, that our team comes together and creates a list of team agreements—how we are going to be with one another. The process of coming to agreement on this list will invariably take time and effort. Then it will probably take an equal effort or more to hold people to the agreement. There is usually very little flexibility surrounding this agreement. In fact, someone is normally appointed to maintain the agreement, which adds another level of effort to the mix. Everyone seems to win, but we still find ourselves working hard to maintain our winning ways. Unfortunately, many people remember the compromises they had to make, and invariably, during the next conversation these points come up. This state of mind can often be found in labor-management negotiations.

The highest level of interaction we see is what we call the alignment model. The skill associated with this level of relationship is the ability to listen at deeper levels. It is not about debate or negotiation. It is about listening for the grains of truth being spoken. The alignment level speaks directly to mindfulness. It's an ability to almost listen in between the words. When people can listen quietly from this state of alignment, their solutions that emerge not only embrace all the grains of truth in all positions, but take our understanding to a higher level. The response is often, "Wow, I didn't see it that way, and that is actually much better than what I see!"

Moving From Adversarial to Alignment

To illustrate this process, let us look at two stories in which organizations moved from the adversarial stage to an alignment model.

We were working with a healthcare systems organization and the senior team was discussing a pending merger and resulting downsizing. The financial group was saying things like, "We have to make ourselves look as good as possible financially to our potential acquirer." The other camp was saying, "That's true, but we cannot turn our backs on our employees because they have all been here for years. So we can't just go out and slash and burn to get our profitability up." They had been talking about this issue for months. They were trying to keep their spirits up, but when they got low, the discussion invariably turned argumentative. They slipped into debate, angrily declaring which one of them was more right.

The financial camp faction would say, "If this merger occurs short-term, we downsize, but long-term we can hire them back." The people faction would counter, "If we whack

our people, they won't want to come back to our company."
They were locked at this level of debate. Realizing they were
getting nowhere fast, and understanding that continuing on
this adversarial level would cause even more disruption, they
raised the conversation to the next stage. Finance offered,
"We'll set aside some money for things like out-placement,
but in return we have to let go of more people." Negotiations
began and give-and-take ensued. "Surely, we can find a win-
win solution here," was the sentiment.

When we came in, our job was to help them listen to one
another. When this started happening, they began hearing
the grains of truth in both positions. Then someone in the
people camp bridged the gap and said, "I wonder if there is a
way if our people could become healthy enough it would create enough of a dramatic impact on the bottom line that it
would provide the solution to what Finance wants to see happen." What they realized was that if the people in the organization were healthy enough, instead of the senior management team having to come up with a solution, the workforce
could develop one. They had gotten stuck in an old model in
which the senior team was supposed to solve these problems.
In this situation, they returned to the level of faith and trust
in the people they hired to come up with a solution, and the
senior team would then be there to guide them.

They went about the task of increasing the health of the
organization with the top 400 people in the organization. All
of these people went through a seminar/workshop that
exposed them to these ideas and to their thinking. Out of
that context, they completely redesigned the paradigms of
management, leadership, and organization, and they made it

happen. It wasn't a win-lose or win-win resolution, but a higher form of winning in which the entire culture benefited without having to waste effort in debate and negotiation. The right solution emerged out of the healthy, aligned interactions of the senior team and then the organization because it was allowed to come from that mindful rather than mind-filled place.

Another example occurred at NYNEX. We began working with an HR group that two days before had received notice that they were going to be disbanded for the sake of a shared-services initiative. The anger and paranoia in the room could be cut with a knife. They were arguing back and forth: "The values of this organization were nothing but a bunch of words. The company lacks integrity." Then one camp emerged that decided it was going to hold the company hostage. The other side decided they just weren't going to work. Knowing they were going to be cut loose, they wouldn't come in, but rather would spend their time looking for another job. This was day one and the debate was all about which side should prevail.

Day two dawned and they got to a level of searching for agreement, albeit a very negative one: "OK, if you guys don't squeal on us, we won't squeal on you. If you cover our butts while we're out looking for a job, we'll feign ignorance in terms of some of the things that you want to do to hold the company hostage." This was not a healthy process.

By the third day, they were getting progressively healthier, and they started listening to one another from the perspective of the grain of truth behind what they were saying. Around lunchtime on the third day, a young man stood up and said,

"I've finally settled down enough to listen to what we are all talking about. I chose the field of HR because I wanted to be of value to people in business. That is what is most important to me. I think that now is a perfect opportunity for us to show our mettle. As frightened and angry as we were two days ago, there are a whole slew of people out there in our company that are probably more frightened and angry than we are. The best thing that we can do as HR professionals is to create an oasis of health for those individuals."

The silence in the room was deafening.

Everyone stopped. The anger visibly dissipated from the faces of the group. Some were moved to tears. The last half of the third day was completely different than the first two and a half days. They quieted down. The conversation took up on a human-to-human level. People began relating that they didn't know why they were so afraid. They'd all switched jobs many times before. It's just an inconvenience to have to look again. Another woman said that she had lost her anger toward the company and could actually see why they were doing what they had to do. She could see and appreciate the "humane" way the company had chosen to deal with them.

In the final three hours, they created a brand new vision for that HR department. They decided they were going to be there, not only for each other, but for the rest of the division of about 10,000 people. And they were true to their word. Their actions stood out so prominently that upper management realized that as a company they would be foolish to let these people go. Of the 35 people in the room those three days, NYNEX actively found positions within the organization for 30 of them. The five others who opted to cash out and leave, did so on their own because they wanted to work part-time or were ready to retire.

Creating Dialogue

What this group had done was move from debate to agreement to alignment. And in being mindful with no other intent than to come from a healthy perspective, they kept their jobs with the organization and improved the lives of those with whom they worked. What they did was to see and let go of their fear and insecurity, listen deeply to one another, and allow common sense to emerge.

As we define them, listening and common sense are both excellent examples of humility and wisdom—a desire to be influenced and a willingness to pursue the grains of truth in a conversation. They are a deepening process of understanding and growth. These situations were resolved because those within the group were able to hold their positions lightly to see how they would evolve; as opposed to taking positions, drawing a line in the sand, and sticking to them. Debate and negotiation in this context are memory-based—clever and compromising, but very one-sided, and often divisive. The thinking is based on the assumption that there is a winner and a loser, rather than seeking the higher ground of mutual satisfaction through aligned interactions. As soon as positions are solidified, we remove them from any further interaction. And in nature when organisms stop interacting within their environment, they die out and evolution ends.

Flexible and aligned interactions require that people engage in real dialogue. By that we mean speaking and listening with real openness and consistency for as long as we can without already knowing the answer, and then exploring ideas using insight as the clue and wisdom as the guide. This allows us to move forward without backsliding.

This may be a difficult approach to take in some organizations when a decision has to be made. We might hear, "That's fine when we have the luxury of time, but we don't have the time for this." We have found that there is always time for dialogue. In fact, aligned interactions create more time and better, more executable decisions because time is not wasted on ego and intransigence. As was evident in the NYNEX story, real dialogue is far less time-intensive than the time spent revisiting issues because alignment has not been achieved.

Healthy Meetings

As might be expected, meetings take on a completely different character in a Mindful Corporation, especially when alignment and dialogue are present. Aligned interactions—not necessarily in which everyone agrees, but in which everyone is moving with the same intent—can only produce an environment for higher levels of understanding and greater wisdom to emerge.

In a mind-filled organization in which there is little alignment, we often have meetings for the sake of meetings, or as John Horne at International® describes, "people scheduling meetings because they don't know what else to do. I think companies waste more time on that than on anything else." Another problem he finds is that meetings in unaligned organizations rarely come to solutions because "there are so many people that can't make a decision without making sure everyone agrees to it. Then it becomes that proverbial camel that started out as a horse that was designed by committee and ended up being a camel."

Meeting Specific

When discussing the thinking behind meetings, it is always interesting to look at the variety of myths and beliefs that surround the purpose and facilitation of these gatherings. Like most myths, there may be a grain of truth in them. They were certainly all conceived for a very good reason. But upon seeing them in black and white, their relevance seems to diminish greatly.

Meeting Myths

- Focus comes with the agenda.
- Once published, never deviate from the agenda.
- People will never be able to be totally "direct" or "honest" in a meeting.
- There can't be trust in a meeting until people have worked together for a long period of time, preferably through tough times.
- Time slots increase efficiency and effectiveness.
- Meetings are separate from/in addition to an impediment to my actual work.
- The more you can pack into an agenda, the more you will get done.
- Starting earlier and staying later is cost-effective and time-efficient.
- Meet during breakfast/lunch/dinner to get more done.
- When tension or conflict occur, roll up your sleeves

and press on.
- It is important for senior leaders to have in-depth operations and tactical discussions in order to keep their fingers on the pulse of the business.

If we were to look at a healthy productive meeting in a mindful organization, we would undoubtedly see people freely sharing their views on the topics under discussion, expressing different opinions, and when appropriate, discussing those opinions. People would feel valued and respected. And when the meeting was over, everyone would know that the action items discussed would be appropriately assigned, *and* even if there wasn't complete agreement with the decision, clear alignment would be reached and the decision would be supported.

Sound like a pipe dream? We've seen healthy, productive meetings such as these happen in all kinds of environments. Within the Mindful Corporation, it is essential that we harness the collective wisdom and expertise of all employees in the healthiest, most effective way. For that reason, we have put together the following list to show what happens when health exists in a meeting. This is not a list to be followed without deviation or as a matter of form. Neither is it a prescription for a healthy meeting. When we slip into that kind of forced-mode thinking, we quickly find ourselves in a mind-filled state. The idea here is that these items provide a context out of which we create and re-create our meeting times to provide the greatest health and productivity. They are a primer of reminders and recommendations. Something we can see. While we can certainly describe healthy interactions, we should not use this list as a set of objectives for behavior. We understand that our normal tendency is to pursue "the right way" of doing things on a very behavioral level. The problem that arises, however, is in spite of doing it the "right way," if the expected doesn't happen, we become judgmental. This sets up a double whammy because the more judgmental people get, the further away from health they wander. We refer to this as becoming unhealthy for all the right reasons. In addition to focusing on behavioral or results avenues, we need to keep our eye on the health of the participants and the feeling of the environment when that happens. That is the touchstone.

With that as a caveat, what follows are the characteristics of healthy meetings.

Characteristics Of Healthy Meetings

Meetings begin with attention being paid to the health of the team so the tone of the meeting will be conducive to an open, trusting environment. There is a sense of settling down and mentally arriving.

Primary attention is given to finding common ground and operating from an atmosphere of alignment as well as a commitment to achieve alignment.

Decisions are made, and stay made, not out of rigidity but because alignment was reached and support was acknowledged.

Views and ideas are expressed openly without self-consciousness or doubt.

People listen attentively while others are talking.

Questions are asked to clarify and to gain deeper understanding.

Participant/supporter behaviors are the norm.

People build on each other's ideas and proposals without concern for ownership.

Disagreement and conflict exist and are expressed and discussed in an atmosphere of respect. People do not feel attacked or undermined.

People are open to the possibility that they can change their minds.

There is a bias for developing a shared understanding of issues, values, behaviors, alternatives, and solutions.

Individuals are aware of their personal impact on the health and effectiveness of the meeting and the team.

People look forward to going to meetings because worthwhile work is conducted productively, flexibly, and creatively in a lighthearted atmosphere.

As problems present themselves, there is a bias toward reflection versus reaction.

People have great patience with each other even in times of perceived urgency.

Visitors to the meeting are welcomed and treated with courtesy and respect.

There is a vitality in meetings that allows for brainstorming and free-flowing thinking, and results in faster, more creative, aligned decisions that are clearly supported by all parties.

Finding a Shared Reality

Within the vast numbers of interactions that take place in every organization; between individuals, departments, and divisions, for every idea offered each person will have his or her own interpretation, representation, and formulation. These all come out of our own subjective separate realities. When we meet, however, we often have to learn to release those interpretations so that we can create dialogue and find a shared, aligned reality. The first step in this process is to be aware of our thoughts after they've crossed our mind and treat them lightly. This means not holding them fast, without flexibility. We need to see thoughts as temporary impostors of reality. To do so, we use our feelings as a gauge, an indicator that points us toward those thoughts. In other words, we don't become tied to the interpretations, representations, or formulations we make, but hold them as if they were nothing more than the light, billowy made-up stuff from which all thoughts derive. To consciously wrestle with thoughts and treat them as sacred makes us immediately self-conscious, robbing us of energy and pulling us out of the moment.

We are trying to create an organization whose boundaries and walls are more permeable than not. New information flows easily in and out. The mind-filled organization is one in which courses for further learning are often mandated. In the mindful organization, the culture is continually migrating toward a greater sense of self-discovery. This is why we are trying to stay away from providing a prescription for healthy action. How-to lists are operationally fine when dealing with mechanical issues, but as soon as we enter into aligning the interactions of humans, any and all rigid systems only produce greater rigidity.

Let's look at insecurity as an example. The world seen through the lens of insecurity can be a frightening, irritating, or confusing place. Unaware of the role that thought plays, individuals will automatically act on the basis of how they see what's going on in their world. For example, they may become sullen and uninviting or rant and yell and become belligerent. In the mindful organization, these temporary outbursts are seen with compassion and an understanding that everyone visits that state on occasion. Through their understanding, they are weatherproofed from the barbs of harshness, and become conscious of their own thinking that can push them, too, in these directions. For those caught up in their momentary thoughts of insecurity and anger, this moment is shortened. Being surrounded by health, the odds are increased that perception will return and humanity will prevail.

TVA's Bill Thompson provides an example of this when he describes a seminar he attended at the Wharton School of Business: "The instructor had everyone take a sheet of paper and draw out what they considered to be the universal organization chart. Everyone became very busy drawing these different organization charts, some with customers, some with employees at the top, and others with executives at the top. After debriefing the group to find out what they had come up with, he told us, 'Let me show you the universal organization chart.' He went up to a flip chart and drew a big circle with the word "me" inside it. 'That is the universal organization chart in operation in corporate America today,' he said. 'It is all about me, and my needs.' The point he was making was that every individual's reality was really based on his or her own needs, and to a certain extent, their insecurity. But that was nothing more than a thought habit. If we can get people attached to a vision, a higher calling, a higher purpose, then people will start to give up that intense desire to view life as if 'It is all about me.' And start to see it as 'I'm here for a grander purpose.' I think alignment flows out of that. If you can get people to leave their own personal desires, intentions, and egos at the door, that is when alignment occurs."

Now, this isn't the way the majority of the business world is wired, but then, for the most part, they are not coming from a place of health. What we find again and again is that most organizations are not set up to operate from a healthy perspective. They tend to approach this whole process from the outside-in, which allows their infrastructure to limit them from seeing their own limitations. They try to fix or avoid the element outside of themselves that they are convinced is the cause of their feelings. The Mindful Corporation is about how we conduct business from a healthy perspective, unrestricted by infrastructure. This doesn't mean that we throw out policies, rules, and routines, but those aren't the primary goals toward which we need to be heading.

Policies, Rules, and Procedures in a Healthy Organization

The focus of this process isn't just on what we are doing, but whether or not people are maintaining their health. If the answer is yes they are, then policies, procedures, and routines will follow along in an equally healthy manner. Rules are often necessary when it comes to communicating the wisdom of the moment, ensuring alignment, and correcting expectations. They are not ends in and of themselves. Too often we focus on the implementation of the rules rather than the spirit and understanding behind them.

Most organizations operate out of a set of models constructed to reflect the principles out of which they want to run their businesses. What an organization actually does, its behaviors, are in constant interaction with the models that have been built. That interaction between model and behavior is constantly evolving. Policies, procedures, and routines are then devised to support the model and guide the behavior. They are only as valid as the model they support. And since our models are constantly changing, our rules and policies need to be flexible as well.

Rules are not intended to generate behavior, but to serve as a guide to provide alignment toward purpose. If rules are seen as hard and fast, dictating behavior, then we have no way of developing beyond them, or creating anything new or novel.

Rules can also take the place of one of the most significant issues within an organization: communication. If we have a rule in place, it frees us from having to communicate our need any more. We simply point to the rule. But the Mindful Corporation is predicated on our ability to communicate in a healthy fashion. As greater wisdom or common sense finds its way into how we do business, the ability to communicate becomes tremendously important instantly. Our capacity to organize the organization depends on it. Form follows philosophy, so the infrastructure of our organizations must remain pliable and open to change. If form leads philosophy, nothing new emerges because we are already coming from a solidified perspective. As an organization grows in size and in location, the complexity of its interactions also increases. However, if more people operate from and in a healthy state of mind, we would find that alignment and optimal functioning occur and a great deal of the complexity actually falls away. When we give people free reign with their wisdom and common sense, the organization naturally evolves in that direction.

Look at the wonderfully crafted documents at the heart of most lasting societies. Regardless of the intent of the forefathers, the documents of those countries tried to capture this spirit—that at any point in time, the organization was both perfect and imperfect. They had the humanity to build into their models the opportunity for change, for decisions to be made from wisdom and dialogue honoring the best that man could be, yet understanding and correcting when he faltered. There are many parallels to this approach for business, as imperfect as it may appear.

Enabling Organization

As we also find in nature, when we operate from a mindful perspective, organization tends to take place. We find evolution and effective self-organization. This comes about not out of some magical wishing it to happen, but because people are aware enough to recognize what is required to move the organization forward. When organizations are aligned in this fashion, it doesn't take external motivation or reward to make things work. Common sense alone dictates what is required, not rules and procedures. Again, this does not happen simply because we want it to, but because we have seen to the health of the individual and organization. In short, it happens because we have created the Mindful Corporation.

Currently, most organizations operate by means of the "bigger hammer" technique. We organize by directive. In doing so, for the sake of control and the illusion of ensuring equanimity, consistency, and comprehension, we limit what is truly possible within the organization as we limit growth. The image we are offering is an organization that, because of its health and wisdom, isn't driven by these outer mechanisms of rules and procedures, but is capable of using them as the tool they were intended to be. We harvest them for the grains of truth and wisdom that went into devising them, and then apply those as required.

Very few people, let alone organizations, are comfortable with the idea of constant evolution. They need plateaus to have a sense of stability. What we do, then, is create these limitations within our processes through which we think we can control the evolution of the organization. If we view these plateaus as temporary rest stops, we don't allow them to impede our organizational growth. Since we all have good days and bad days, the plateaus might be seen as nothing more than healthy spots for us to spend our bad days. If we, however, solidify these resting spots into concrete bunkers in which we hunker down, we dramatically slow and limit our evolution to the point where extinction is usually not too far away. Nature is actually fine when systems die. Business, however, and its investors are usually not as comfortable with it.

Why do our organizations need to become more mindful? Without the health of the people, the "leader-led organization" becomes mandatory. Once we can make health a commodity, then this process of self-organization and leadership-via-wisdom that we are describing will become a reality. If health is only experienced by a chosen few within the company, then the present model will just continue.

However, if we assemble a business of healthy individuals who understand the principles we've been discussing, in very short order, people outside the organization will point to us and ask, "How the heck are they doing what they are doing?" The answer will not be the structure, system, strategy, or any business initiative, but it will be the organization's nurturing and attention to the health of its people.

Chapter Eight

Boundaryless Coaching

"Ego is promoting our own personal reality as if it
were all there is."

—

Dicken Betinger

One characteristic that has marked human development is that
we are always ready and willing to share what we know with
others. Sometimes we do so when it may not be wanted, and
other times when we only understand part of the picture. Still,
we are compelled to offer our knowledge.

We often deliver this seemingly altruistic gift in the same
fashion that we learned from our parents and teachers, and
yet we are surprised when we are met with a similar effect—
dismissal. But as the Broadway musical composer Stephen
Sondheim once noted in song, "No matter what you say, children will listen." In spite of our occasional wish to blot out
what someone may be trying to teach us, we hear what is said.
When two living beings interact, something different always
emerges out of that interaction. This is called co-evolution, in

which both parties evolve as a product of their interaction. This idea is not new. Recorded discussions of co-evolution in India date back over 2500 years, but the recent studies of emergence have brought it forward again.

What we see, however, is that if that interaction takes place when both parties are locked in memory and forced mode, all that emerges is more of the same. But when both people interact in flow mode, new vistas open up that neither person may have anticipated. Invariably, in these instances, the environment created by the interaction provides the space for one of the people involved to have an insight and pass through a doorway of understanding. That insight is not created by the interaction, but it certainly helped put both people at the bus stop ready to be picked up. At this point of insight, a uniquely human attribute occurs. The person who has had the insight has an opportunity to turn to his or her companion and offer them entree into this new space on the other side of the threshold of understanding. If that person accepts, the two move toward the next threshold. If there is a refusal for any reason, whether because of insecurity or fear, that person is left behind. Often, strain in relationships can arise when one person moves through succeeding doorways while the other continually stays back. Our natural inclination, however, is to help the other to move across the threshold. We have found that in this coaching process, all we can do is help co-create the environment at the doorway so that the co-evolutionary process can take place. Each step taken is up to the individual.

There are still some leaders in organizations who don't think that coaching applies to them. Tiger Woods is one example that Bill Thompson at TVA applies to those who are reluctant to accept coaching. Without question the greatest golfer of this era, Thompson reminds us that, "Woods has a personal coach. He knows that as good as he is he needs to get better. The guy who is coaching him is not the best golfer in the world, but yet Tiger is open to listening to an independent point of view and incorporating it into his approach to the game. When we get into the board rooms of corporate America, for some reason, that superstar, willingness-to-improve mentality goes away. Our corporate executives have convinced themselves that they are in that board room because they are swell. The notion that they can do even better is somehow foreign to them. The behavioral norm is an ego thing. 'I'm who I am and I am wonderful and I don't need to work on stuff to get even better.' What they don't understand is how self-limiting their own thinking is. If we can create a culture where folks actually want coaching, where they feel comfortable asking, 'How can I do even better?' and receiving that reply from whoever makes sense to them, we create a very powerful, competitive weapon for any company."

Coaching and Coaches

We have found that in this world of boundaryless coaching, through their interaction, both parties are changing and, in turn, changing each other. The assumption that the coachee is the one changing and the coach remains the same is simply not true. We have been taught to differentiate between the role of coach and coachee, but the process of co-evolution won't allow it. It speaks directly to the relationship at hand, not necessarily to the roles of those relating. We have focused primarily on the person being coached, what he or she is hearing, and the resultant change in behavior. After the fact, when we talk to the coach, we find that the more successful coaches learn a great deal from the coaching experience. This is true for managers, teachers, and leaders as well.

Because the coaching process involves the interactions of two or more people, it is anything but linear. It does not progress neatly from point to point in a prescribed or expected sequence. When we have choices to make, we do so from an unlimited array of adjacent possibilities. These possibilities exist one thought away from actualization, just waiting to be recognized. Whenever we make a choice, we create a whole new realm of adjacent possibilities. In essence, they represent a never-ending envelope of potential. In forced mode, however, we often limit and narrow those choices to what we already know, and in so doing miss out on some unexpected possibilities or those that, perhaps, are inconceivable within our current prospective.

Within a flow state, we have access to all the possibilities.

Picking the Ripe Possibility

We might compare these possibilities to an apple tree filled with ripening apples. The nonlinear apples are not neatly spaced throughout the tree. We have lots of choices available as to which we pick, but sometimes, as was true in Newton's case, we simply wait until one falls on our head. This is because, as we mentioned earlier, the operative word in this emergent insight process is "unexpected." The idea is to remain in a humble, curious state, and like Newton, see what bonks us on the head. In a mindful, boundaryless coaching process, we are not looking for any one thing.

As we introduced in the previous chapter, coaching is about creating rapport and alignment. And here, too, the three "A's"—adversarial, agreement, and alignment—indicate the three tiers that differentiate the levels of coaching. In alignment, a higher level of co-evolution is achieved than is possible by any one party involved. Instead of compromise or collaboration, we reach a level of synergy that transcends and embraces both positions totally. Both alignment and rapport depend heavily on the state of healthy and deep listening. Without rapport (respect, trust, and faith), the listeners have difficulty staying in this state of humility—truly open to being influenced by the other party's grains of truth.

Three Levels of Coaching

When coaching from the lower adversarial state, the skill employed is argument and debate. This kind of coaching becomes an exercise in power and influence. The influence is extended by the one who is "perceived" as the winner in the conversation. It is very much a win-lose type of relationship. This is a coaching relationship based on authority and memory, and consequently, there is very little novel co-evolution taking place.

Often, people who have recently joined an organization feel themselves in this position: "First learn the way *we* play the game, and then you can think on your own." To a large extent, the determining factor in an adversarial coaching relationship is fatigue. People give up. They separate from this coaching relationship feeling less than fulfilled. There is a high degree of coercion in the relationship and no rapport. There is also rarely a buy-in by the coachee. The only shift in behavior we might see is out of compliance rather than commitment. It is based on the traditional roles of coach and coachee, not interaction and exchange.

The next "A" of coaching is agreement, and the skill here is negotiation. How can we compromise? While it does appear to be a win-win situation, we are involved in compromise, which translates into "I'll give up something if you give up something." When we find what we are willing to give up, we also discover what we are willing to build upon. This is a lot better than adversarial coaching because people leave in a better state of mind, but they don't leave as if they have completely won. The consequences of this approach are that the "seeds of discontent" are often planted at the moment of agreement, only to bare fruit further down the road. Instead of building closer relationships, we sow the seeds of greater negotiation. In the short term, people shake hands and part company, not as adversaries but not as functional co-workers either. Often, there is still a feeling of an amicable "us and them."

The next level of coaching is alignment. The skill here is deep listening. This is the home of boundaryless coaching, the space out of which our healthy interactions allow for the greatest insight; that is, the state of being open to unexpected adjacent possibilities. In this state of conversation, the solution appears and embraces all the grains of truth in all positions. It takes us to a higher level of seeing. When we coach in a state of alignment, our reality shifts. In the first two approaches, reality doesn't shift. All we are doing is rearranging the deck chairs. But in a state of alignment, we are listening for insight. When we hear it, our reality shifts and we cross the threshold into a whole new understanding.

In the alignment state, rapport aligns the interaction and readies the environment for insight to happen. Our rapport in the agreement state simply allows the conversation to occur.

Ron Adams tells a story of two instances that cross a number of these levels. He first had to produce a product for a leader with whom he had an adversarial relationship. When Ron delivered the product, he received dictatorial and harsh feedback, which he didn't agree with it. It then took a tremendous amount of energy for him to make the demanded corrections. During the whole process, he was mad and frustrated and he delivered changes that were just barely acceptable.

In the second instance, with another leader, Adams describes, "I didn't agree with the needed changes, but because of the respect and rapport I had with him, I assumed he was right. My number one goal was not the product, but to re-establish rapport with the coach. I gave it 120 percent of my attention and I became even closer with the coach. The business case was the same, the product was the same, but the difference was the rapport."

Building rapport begins with a state of mind in which we find ourselves truly curious about the other person and open to being touched by their spirit and world. When two people are in this state of rapport and good will, judgments and impatience fall away. We find ourselves listening to more than just the words—the content of the conversation—but to the entire person. The outcome of this state of mind is that healthy working relationships are initiated. We become aware when our personal thoughts are interfering with our more transcendent thoughts.

We believe this state of rapport is one of our default innate states that provides a sense of peace and relaxation. When we find ourselves outside of these states, we have been taught to go forward nonetheless, and forcibly re-create it if necessary. In a well-meaning attempt to do so, some people turn to outside influences—alcohol, exercise, vacations—to re-create the state of relaxation and peace. The truth of the matter is, to a certain degree we've all bought the idea we can force it and bring it about. And as soon as we enter into re-creating these states, we introduce stress and effort to our lives.

The Rapport of Children at Play

The alternative to re-creating these states when we've slipped out of them is to calm our thoughts. This could take the form of a moment or two of quiet reflection, going for a walk, or simply taking a break. We find that when we recognize where our thinking has taken us, we automatically return to our natural state. The easiest place to see this in action is to watch children. Kids who have never met come together on the playground, and they are immediately in a state of rapport. It is not because of what they do; it is because of where they come from. That "come from" is an uncontaminated, innate state. How they act is based on rapport.

This is not a case, however, of doing. We don't *do* rapport. We are simply in a state of rapport. As we have mentioned earlier, we are relating beings. All we have is our ability to perceive and relate. When our perception is off, our relating is off. When perception is stuck in outmoded memory or in feelings that indicate lower levels of understanding, don't push forward—cool out for a short while. We all need a quiet space sometimes. We can guarantee that during this time the world will not pass us by. This time-out allows us to integrate our thoughts and align them naturally so we can return and operate again from a state of rapport.

Why is this important? Because there is a direct link between the amount of rapport we have and what we can get done in a healthy way. When people are in rapport, there is much more listening and finding ways to make things work, and less rigidity to the way it is or needs to be. We also find that there is more good will. We are more ready to give people the benefit of the doubt, to forgive them, and find synergy between us. If our organizations exhibited these traits and characteristics, wouldn't any task be much easier and happen more quickly? We think so.

When we are in rapport together, we can find ways of dealing with issues and problems in a more healthy fashion because we don't have all the layers of doubt and mistrust that keep us from the task at hand. And when someone with an agenda pops up, we can see its innocence—its momentary thought—often even before the person with the agenda sees it, and not take it personally. We simply wait for the other person to regain their bearings.

Sometimes, however, even mindful leaders revert. What happens for Larry Senn is that "if I have neglected someone for a period of time and am not aware of what they have been doing and/or I haven't commented on contributions that they have made, and then I just come at them out of the blue with something I don't like, they get really defensive. The little voice comes back saying, 'but don't you know that I did "a," "b" and "c," and you never said anything about that. How come you are only talking to me about "d?" '"

It is not always easy to get to this place of recognizing thoughts while they happen. The important factor is that they are recognized, whether an hour later, a day, or a year. Even if we miss it entirely, we'll undoubtedly have other opportunities. That is one thing life always affords us; plenty of opportunities to deal with sharp edges. If we remain conscious of them, sooner or later we'll learn.

The Intent of the Listener

This is one of the great benefits of boundaryless coaching. If we are capable of listening with the true intent of being influenced by the other person—with true curiosity and without judgment—we enable the speaker to speak with less agenda and anticipation. In coaching situations like these, the persons talking feel the coaches are not only on their side, but want to provide them with the best and gentlest situation for insight to arise and facilitate their learning. There is a "flow" of unprejudiced words that allows them to reflect on their thinking. At this point, the subtleties, and sometimes not so subtle clues, can appear for the speakers, leading them to the thought-source of why they are seeking coaching. The beauty is that persons being coached in this fashion are less defensive and more open to seeing their thinking in this state. Frequently, the insights occur to the speakers before the coaches can say anything. On more than one occasion we have heard, "The coach didn't tell me anything, I discovered it all myself."

The technique is simple. If we want to appear like a genius, we need to surround ourselves with excellent listeners. Ego and insecurity aside—yes-men need not apply—an excellent listener makes it easier for a person to get into a flow state. If the intent of coaching is to bring out the best in others and improve their performance, then the key is to be a good listener.

The subtle clues that allow us to gain a clear perspective of our behaviors don't come when a person is yelling at us. How many times have we received obvious coaching and then kept getting the same obvious coaching year after year after year? What is helpful are the not-so-obvious clues that are, in fact, life-altering. These clues may be an innocuous observation someone makes about the manner in which we had spoken to another. Suddenly a ray of light shines onto a thought pattern we'd never recognized before. When these moments emerge, there is an immediate "Whoa!" What bowls us over is the implication of the moment of truth, not the content of the insight.

Coaching is necessary because we are all human. There is always something too close to home for us to step away from. Even as we evolve, we will feel "off" our game, confused or insecure. We will perceive life as something that pushes on us at the right moment to cause some degree of insecurity. As we become more attuned to our flow state, this insecurity is less intense and remains with us for shorter periods of time. But every now and then it pops up, and that is the time we need a coach.

Creating the Environment for Insight

Boundaryless coaching creates the environment; it lays the groundwork that facilitates insight. The key here is that insight doesn't come from the environment, it comes out of us and is actually not contingent upon what is happening around us, but on our state of mind.

This takes us back to the opening of this chapter when we were discussing interactions out of which something transcendent emerges. Our aligned interactions create the environment that carries with it all the attendant positive traits of alignment, but the emergence itself is personal.

Within the coaching interaction, we become aware as we approach an emergent state. Someone might say something with a grain of truth that is just enough to trigger us, and the insight emerges. It might appear that the interaction caused the insight, but it did not. The insight is not contingent on any action we take. Its potential is always ready and waiting for us to cross the threshold and realize it. All the interaction did was bring us to the doorway of what was possible.

Suppose, for instance, we are in a very insightful, quiet flow state when we jog, and we associate our jogging with being in that state. The moment we do that we limit our possibilities of finding that state when doing something else. Being in a state of mindfulness has nothing to do with what we do. But what we do has everything to do with our state of mindfulness.

The greater degree to which we can understand that, the less likely we will be knocked off our feet when people don't act the way we expect. When we view the world inside-out, relating is a function of our state of mind. In an outside-in world, we think our state of mind is a function of our relationships. This understanding is at the heart of building the Mindful Corporation, and the key to the notion of boundaryless coaching.

If we can listen to someone in such a way that it creates an environment from which they can cross over into a mindful state, we have accomplished all we could ever hope as a coach. If the coach tries to give an insight to a coachee, nothing is realized because the person being coached has not moved through the doorway. But if we could continually create environments within our organizations from which we could take each other through succeeding doorways of understanding, what a remarkable powerhouse we would create!

Chapter Nine

Mindful Business

"No one can take from us the joy of first becoming aware of
something, the so-called discovery. But if we also demand
the honor, it can be utterly spoiled for us, for we are usually
not the first. What does discovery mean, and who can say
that he has discovered this or that? After all, it's pure idiocy
to brag about priority, for it's simply unconscious conceit,
not to admit frankly that one is a plagiarist."

—

Goethe

Healing, wisdom, and perspective come from the realization
that thought is illusory, created by us in the moment. In recognizing this, we are also acknowledging that there is a state
from which original thought emerges—a state that exists
before the content of thought or what we think. We have
called this pre-thought, flow, the zone, the here and now.
This is also the mindful state—a state of connectivity
between a more universal, transcendent intelligence and us.

For many of us, this concept turns what we have been
taught topsy-turvy. The idea many have always believed to be

true is that "This is the way good people act." We then attempt to act that way, regardless of whether or not it's how we really see the world. We are suggesting something quite different— that it is more natural for us to be in a healthy state out of which good people act, and then allow our actions to follow.

Here is one aspect of this concept that immediately increases productivity. If the content of our thinking is made up, why spend the time and effort on trying to fix what is illusory? George Pransky likened this to trying to fix a mirage. Why drain something that doesn't exist? This also recalls the difference between imagination and perception that we spoke about earlier. Many of the personal growth groups and movements that sprang up in the latter part of the twentieth century were based on providing ways for us to change the content of our thinking. They provided plenty of techniques and affirmations to alter content for either what we imagined or perceived.

What we are pointing toward precedes that, and as such, is as old as the earliest philosopher. We're talking about the state of pre-thought, from which seeing the process of thought and the role it plays is evident. The state of pre-thought enables us to see the innocence around us. In other words, we are all acting out of how we perceive. For the most part, people act and react out of forced mode or processed memory. They are not doing so because they are bad or good people, but because that's how they've learned to see life. When we see the innocence in others, we are mindful of this and can therefore look for the grain of truth in what they say, but not get personally caught up in their emotions, feelings, or lower states of understanding. When we are able to relate in this fashion, we are seeing the process of thought and its connection to content, actions, and feelings. Innocence does not come from what we think, but from the perspective *that* we think. We can be touched by the state of the healing potential we see in others. We are not trying to teach people how to think, only that in letting go of thought, of not investing in it so much that our thoughts become solid, we can return to that innate state existing in all of us.

Thought-beings

Ever since Rene Descartes, western thinking has been predicated on the idea "I think, therefore I am." But perhaps we should rework this statement to say, "I am, therefore I think."

It is incredibly important for leaders, both for themselves and their corporations, to see the innate health in themselves and those around them. If they can't see this, they and their organizations achieve little learning. Seeing innocence in others also becomes evident in the way we deal with customers. When a leader comes from a healthy, mindful perspective, he or she casts a broad and positive shadow through the organization. People feel energized, included, and invigorated by it. They become inspired, hopeful, and because they are healthier, more resilient to life's challenges. They therefore translate that directly into their encounters with customers. At McDonald's, the implementation of these simple ideas into the restaurants not only improved customer satisfaction and ultimately sales, but according to surveys, also improved the taste of the food; such is the power of innate health.

We should note that seeing the innocence in others does not mean condoning whatever happens. We are suggesting that if changes are needed that they be made, but that they come from healthier, more effective perspectives.

When our leaders are able to see and incorporate the innate health of the people they work with, they don't limit the inspiration and energy of their work force. Decisions are made that defy logic, but yet yield remarkable results. Why? Because the thinking that produced the decisions was not from some standard level of acceptance; it emerged and was recognized from a deeper level of understanding that was more in touch with our natural way of operating.

Making Mindful Choices

Suppose our company is going through a merger in which it has become imperative to downsize. The "normal" and logical way of letting people go would be to create an infrastructure around them so they are protected from hurting themselves and/or the corporation. We would first eliminate their access to computer systems and participation in decision making. We would then set up a separation package or career-counseling program to help them transit this change. That would be the logical approach.

The CEO of Michigan Capital had a different approach. He brought all the people together to get in touch with their own inner strengths and health. Then he included them in every step of the conversation regarding the merger. Once people were in a state of health, he kept them in the loop and involved. As the company went through the downsizing, the CEO didn't have to make harsh or painful decisions. When one of the transition subcommittees got insecure and circled the wagons, making decisions from protect mode, the other subcommittees gently pointed out, "What's your state of mind? What does this reflect as a state of mind?" They all agreed that now was not the time to go down the path of self-rejection, the "looking out for number one" mentality.

Because of these steps, the merger went tremendously smoothly. And of the employees who were involved, about one-third left the company and half of those continued to work for the company on a consulting basis. Good will was retained as was the health and values of the company. Had they approached this from a lower state of understanding, few, if any, would have returned and the company would have been diminished by the impact.

It was all in how they arranged it. Because they approached the situation in a healthy, mindful perspective, there was no sense of loss or separation. This is not sugar-coating something to make it more appealing. That's an outside-in approach, and the effects of that are temporary, at best. This was a process of people's health improving so that they saw life inside-out, and that perspective changes everything. There were the occasional insecure moments, but those were a handful out of hundreds. It was one of the healthiest mergers and downsizings we have ever seen. In spite of that, we can't say, "Do these 10 things in sequence to effect a healthy merger." Human interaction is a very fluid process, but if we have any designs on improving it, we need to start with a program that introduces people to their health.

Like Water Over Obstacles

When we see life as innately healthy, business changes dramatically. When we operate in flow mode, we can see our health as well as the health of those with whom we work. The journey is easier and more hopeful. While the image may seem overused, the process is like a flowing river. A river doesn't focus on overcoming obstacles, it keeps its course and flows over and around any obstacles it encounters. It never says, "If only we could move that rock out of the way. Wouldn't that make life easier?" The river couldn't care less. Its sole purpose is to continue its flow.

What would our business look like if the thinking that creates our obstacles suddenly dissolved as the illusion it is? Like the river, we would simply flow, heedless of rapids or falls, stopped only by the dams constructed with our own thoughts. This is why we believe that while ambitious, the Mindful Corporation may be the best way to bring this understanding into the world. The company that embraces this way of doing business will have healthier individuals who create improved performance relationships between themselves and within their industries.

By developing physically, mentally, emotionally, and spiritually healthier ways of doing profitable business, we have a greater positive impact on the world around us. This is not a pipe-dream scenario that is impossible to enact, let alone envision. This is our innate natural way of living in the world. If these are our normal default settings, then doing business in this fashion is also the normal way of doing business. This is an archetypal approach to life in its original form. What we are suggesting is a return to the state before rules of business were invented. When we come from our innate way of living in the world, we provide an equally natural and harmonious way of doing business. The root source of stress and tension in business comes from our fighting our natural tendencies of health.

What would industry have to do to capture all the benefits that we have spelled out in this book? First, we need to have patience with this understanding. We need to focus on our strategies while being aware of the feeling of health in all that we do. The fact is, we can only set the stage. We can't guarantee a person will experience greater health, or see life through insight, or even be touched by its grandeur. We simply cannot force results and behaviors in anyone's life or in our own.

It's About Allowance Not Force

The process of the Mindful Corporation is about allowing philosophy in rather than driving a philosophy through. Industry needs to recognize that place of allowance. That is hard for business because it has always operated out of a push mentality, and decades of push have done more harm than good. It's not that business doesn't occasionally realize this. The Just-in-Time introduction in the mid-1980s brought in a whole philosophy of pull rather than push, allowing us to pull product when it was needed rather than have it pushed onto us through the supply chain. But then we went through a cycle of reengineering and downsizing, pushing out and restructuring in our zeal to pull organizations forward faster. But all of a sudden, organizations realized that there was no life or spirit left in their companies. They were lean, but they were no longer alive. So a short period of allowance took hold in which we heard, "OK, we have to heal now." Then, once that health started to return, the very philosophy that caused the problem in the first place returned. Suddenly, we're swimming with the sharks again. The thinking in business has been that a little bit of health goes a long way. Very few people have been able to see the wisdom of holding to health. Now that business is changing over to Internet speed, we have to find better ways of dealing with the vast complexity of information and input, of relationships and alliances. That is why the need for health and the practice of the Mindful Corporation have emerged. The ultimate Just-in-Time is really "Be here now." We have found that it's hard to implement a Just-in-Time philosophy with an insecure mentality. The telltale signs are always stress and tension. There are organizations that have embraced Just-in-Time, but have created more stress and tension in their organizations than there was before. That is because they have tried to implement a system without the wisdom to do it.

A crucial dimension of the Mindful Corporation is our humility, that we don't have to have an immediate answer and the issues at hand have nothing to do with us (ego), but rather having understanding and knowledge of a transcendent wisdom greater than our own.

Unless we have confidence in the moment and the wisdom it can provide, Just-in-Time, in any formulation, becomes marginal because the system has very little anticipation, preparation, or stockpiling built in. This process has always required excellent vendor relations and communications. Imagine what would happen if both customers and suppliers throughout the supply chain were coming from a mindful perspective....

A New Viewpoint on Business

We would no longer protect and defend the product of our thinking. We would embrace the philosophy that the product of our thinking was not something we laid claim to or owned. We would maintain separate companies depending on the focus of where we applied our wisdom, but we could actually multiply our effectiveness exponentially by truly partnering with one another rather than spending billions protecting our products.

We are suggesting that when two Mindful Corporations interact in an aligned fashion, we have a boundaryless cooperative interchange. We are not saying it is easy to get beyond the ownership of ideas. It is not. That is the importance of the quote by Goethe that opened this chapter. To see credit for what we devise in a healthy and neutral way goes against a lot of ingrained insecurity we have made up.

It all returns to the quality of our thinking. And in this era of intellectual capital, we find ourselves constrained by our own cleverness. How do we help people become more secure in the fact that by letting go of their proprietary natures, they are not letting go of all the things that make them a business? Few, if any, in business have probably ever done this. For most companies, one great idea is made to last 20 years, and they will defend their proprietary nature to the death. The thinking is obviously that the insight was special, the effort that went into proving it expensive, and there is the possibility that they will never again have another good idea quite like it.

There is another way of doing this while still being able to realize financial and business success. But it can only take place when we focus on mindfulness and not the product of our thinking. When we don't do this, we begin to divide turf, and walls go up. Ownership stifles growth. We fail to see that our thoughts are nothing more than the artifact of our state of mind. We are not pointing toward the quality of the thought or product, but the state of mindfulness out of which it emerged.

As mentioned earlier, we get stuck in proprietary ideas, often because we fear we'll never have another good idea. We become too focused on the product, not the state from which the product was born. If we knew we were an endless source of new ideas, we might view this differently. Every idea would not need to be exploited to its maximum. It has been said that if Albert Einstein, who many consider to be *the* man of the twentieth century, had become a corporation based on his ideas, he would be the largest corporation in the world today. His ideas led directly to the invention of such products as photoelectric cells, TV cameras and televisions, optical sound tracks for movies, devices that carry telephone calls over fiber-optic cables, solid-state devices like calculators and computers, drugs produced via the fusion process, lasers and, consequently, bar-code scanners, power generators, precision clocks—and the list goes on. Had he chosen to keep these ideas proprietary, the world would be far different, and he would never have become "man of the century."

An Idea-rich Environment

Maintaining an idea-rich environment and one constantly open to new ideas is going to be essential as the Boomer generation retires and the X-gen, Net-Gen come into their own. With more jobs than people to fill them, the Mindful Corporation will be able to attract these younger players much more easily than those organizations in which ideas are shielded and systems are closed. The fabric of the Mindful Corporation will enable people to think their best thoughts, prioritize effectively, make laser-quick decisions, and create healthy, high-performance relationships.

In addition, with more to do and less people to do it, there will be a heavy reliance on changing technology. And with all the added tension and stress created by the challenges of increased workloads, it's going to bring out the best and worst in people and their companies. People in demand are going to be lured by greater perks, increased pay, more benefits, and flexible jobs. And the "cool" factor, which is so powerful today, will subside as the Net Generation ages. We will also be seeing a greater divide between the "haves" and the "have nots." The invisible dimension that is going to make the difference in who works where and for whom will be the nature of the fabric of the culture of the company, not its design. Mindfulness, and its attention to awareness and consciousness, will become the key that will satisfy these creative minds.

At a certain point, an organization can only offer so many tangible incentives to lure employees. Today, we're seeing enticements and perks—like getting to drive a sports car—if hired to work for a certain organization. One person we know who has worked for a small software company in Silicon Valley, got to the point, after five years of jumping from company to company, where he realized that the difference between pay, perks, hours, and the prettiness of an office was very small. What became important at that point was the quality of the culture. It's his belief that in Silicon Valley—which could very well be a microcosm of tomorrow—the dimension that will determine where people work and where they apply their genius is going to be an invisible one that can't be captured by a pay scale or even a car.

Recognizing the Wheat and the Chaff

The more mindful an organization becomes, the more likely it will attract and retain healthy and innovative people. And as that healthy awareness takes hold, we will also see a change in the very nature of competition. Health is our inner state of mind. Competition is either an external event or how we think of that external stimulus. How we respond to that outer force will be determined by our health as an organization. On the basis of health, we will be better able to perceive possible threats or dangers as real or imaginary. We will recognize the urgency of a situation and recognize that our appropriate actions are not based on habit or a knee-jerk reaction but are based upon a healthy perspective and the accompanying wisdom. In fact, we have seen situations in which two competitors in a state of health merge to provide a greater service at a better price, as partners rather than as adversaries. Now, this may be the foundation of thought behind mergers and acquisitions, but two organizations' ability to pull it off is purely a function of their health and leadership, and nothing else. Without health in an organization, there can be no sustained, aligned interactions. These two competitors operating out of a state of health no longer saw themselves as an outside-in threat—"the competition"—but were able to align as partners. Competition is an illusion. If we are providing quality and service in the marketplace, it doesn't matter who our competitors are, and there is no need to waste time draining the mirage.

The key to doing things better and optimizing profit is doing them in health rather than through insecurity, anger, tension, or with a stress-driven, fearful environment.

Better operations and greater profits are goals just like anything else; we can pursue them in a fashion that is either healthy or unhealthy. The goals of the Mindful Corporation are greater than simply adding shareholder value. Business is in a unique position to actually help pave the way for a more mindful society because it is moving toward the embodiment of all dimensions of secular life.

J. Krishnamurti once said, "Society is the relationship between you and me and if our relationship is based on ambition, each one of us wanting to be more powerful than the other, then obviously we shall always be in conflict. Where there is fear, there is no intelligence. To live is to find out for yourself what is true. You can do this only when there is freedom, when there is continuous revolution inwardly within yourself."

There is no laying claim to what we, as humans, encounter. All we can do is access the wisdom available to us all. It's like the example used earlier—the planet Pluto was out in space long before we ever discovered it, and our discovery didn't change it a bit. The wisdom is all around us. We are not the only ones to have heard it or thought it, or accessed it. It's simply there for the enabling. The Mindful Corporation only requires our ability to recognize its potential and to enter its flow.

Index

A

Abdoo, Dick, 50-51
accepting ambiguity, 15-16
accountability, 51-52, 122
Adams, Ron, 28, 47, 65, 144, 171
adaptability, 119
adversarial organizations, 146, 148-50
adversarial state, and coaching, 169
agreement, in coaching, 170
Alice in Wonderland, 83
alignment model, 147-48, 152-53, 160
  co-evolution, 169
  in coaching, 170-71
allowance, recognizing place of, 185-86
ambition, 102
answers
  levels of thinking, 112
  looking for, 7
  quieting your mind, 110
  slowing down for perspective, 94
  waiting in humility for, 16
Apple Computers, 44
arrogance
  better than someone else, 101
  state of knowing, 100
Arthur, Brian, 80
awareness
  Being Here Now, 48-52
  level of, 11

B

Bailey, Joseph, 103, 106
balance, work-life, 97
banking, 76-78
Banks, Sidney, 53
bare attention, 107
"Be Here Now" orientation, 48-52
beginner's mind, xxii, 1
behavioral statements, 125-26
beliefs, feelings, and convictions, 86-89
Berra, Yogi, 116
Best, Bob, 26, 47, 119-20, 144
best thinking, policies and procedures as, 40-42

Betinger, Dicken, 165
bigger hammer technique, 163
black sheep, 45-46
  behavior, 46
bliss, following your, 105
boredom, 94
bottom line
  healthy perspective, 191
  leadership prerogatives, 117-18
  mergers, 120
  mindful approach, 80-81
  results-driven orientation, 48, 88
boundaryless coaching, 170-71, 174
boundaryless cooperative exchange, 187
British Telecom (BT), 37-38
Brown, John Seely, 139
bucket of sweat syndrome, 91-92
Buddhists, 107
burnout, 5-7
  coping with symptoms, 6-7
  crisis motivation, 5-6

C

cadences, 84
calmness in activity, 94
Campbell, Joseph, 105
Carlson, Richard, 103, 106, 110
Champy, James, 80, 114
change
  approaches to, 9-10
  humility and, 130
  mind-filled thinking, 17-18
  pace of, 18
  resiliency, 50
  risk of loss, xxi
Childress, John R., 23
Chodron, Pema, 79
choice, 168-69
clarity, 19
co-evolution, 165-66
  coaching process, 167-68
coachees, listening and insight, 174-75
coaching, 36-37
  boundaryless, 170-71, 174

About
Senn-Delaney Leadership

The Senn-Delaney Leadership Consulting Group was founded in 1978 with a specific mission: Assist CEOs and senior executives to create High-performance Teams and Winning Cultures. Today, Senn-Delaney Leadership is a global firm known for its experience and accomplishments in the areas of Culture-Shaping, Teambuilding and Leadership Development. While management consultants work on formulating strategy, structure, systems, and processes, we as leadership consultants focus on creating the organizational and team effectiveness needed to ensure those change initiatives work.

High-performance teams and winning cultures are of utmost importance today. Research and experience confirm that the shortfall in most change initiatives is due to the human issues, not the technical ones. This is true for mergers, new leaders, new strategies, restructures, IT installations and all other major changes.

For over 20 years, we've worked with corporate leaders in the Energy, Information Technology, Financial Services, and Consumer Products/Diversified industries. Our clients include: Agilent, Toys "R" Us, Bell Atlantic, Pacific Bell, Sprint, British Telecom, British Gas, Commonwealth Edison, Portland General Electric, Florida Power and Light, Compaq Computer, IBM PC Division, Hewlett Packard, McDonald's U.S., PepsiCo, Bank One, GTE Information Services and Rockwell International. We have also aided the merger and acquisition transition process within organizational recombinations such as: Chemical-Chase Bank, Ohio Edison-Centerion, Southwestern Bell-Pacific Bell Directory, Compaq-Digital, and Bank One, First Chicago, and National Bank of Detroit.

As we enter the new millennium, the professionals of the Senn-Delaney Leadership Consulting Group remain committed to our vision of "Making a Difference Through Leadership™."

For additional information about the consulting services of Senn-Delaney Leadership, please visit our website at: www.senndelaneyleadership.com.

SENN-DELANEY LEADERSHIP
Part of the Provant Solution
3780 Kilroy Airport Way, Long Beach, CA 90806
Phone (562) 426-5400
Fax (562) 426-5174

www.ingramcontent.com/pod-product-compliance
Lightning Source LLC
Chambersburg PA
CBHW071051280326
41928CB00050B/2170